Praise for Dr. Mark Thompson

"Dr. Thompson is an Alfred Kinsey for the Internet age."

—Philip Zimbardo, PhD, professor of psychology at Stanford University, former president of the American Psychological Association, bestselling author of *The Lucifer Effect*

"Dr. Thompson is a matchmaking genius."

—Michael Georgeff, PhD, former director of the Stanford Artificial Intelligence Institute

WHO SHOULD YOU HAVE SEX WITH?

WHO SHOULD YOU HAVE *Sex* WITH?

THE SECRETS TO GREAT SEXUAL CHEMISTRY

DR. MARK THOMPSON

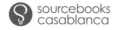
sourcebooks
casablanca

Published by Sourcebooks Casablanca, an imprint of Sourcebooks, Inc.
P.O. Box 4410, Naperville, Illinois 60567-4410
(630) 961-3900
Fax: (630) 961-2168
www.sourcebooks.com

Library of Congress Cataloging-in-Publication Data

Thompson, Mark G. (Mark Gregory)
  Who should you have sex with? : the secrets to great sexual chemistry / by Mark Thompson.
    p. cm.
Includes bibliographical references.
1. Sex instruction. 2. Sex (Psychology) I. Title.
HQ31.T47 2010
613.9'6--dc22
                    2010014372

Printed and bound in the United States of America.
VP 10 9 8 7 6 5 4 3 2 1

Contents

Acknowledgments

The research featured in this book was made possible by the intelligence, hard work, and dedication of many colleagues, collaborators, and research assistants. I am extraordinarily indebted to my longtime friend and research collaborator Glenn Hutchinson, who shaped my thinking on personality, compatibility, and relationships in a profound and lasting way. I would like to thank my friend and business partner Jim Corzine for sticking by my side through thick and thin and for being my trusted ally in battling corporate villains. I am also grateful for the exceptional skills and good humor that Jon Spiller brought in championing many of the studies in this book. Thanks also to Tony Aly, Mary Baker, Peggy Beardeslee, Cecile Conn, Alan Dennis, Michael Georgeff, Jeff Jacka, Wendy Jung, and Philip Zimbardo for their many technical and scientific contributions to this body of research.

Special thanks to my parents, Joel and Dianne Thompson, for lending me their cabin and bringing me care packages while I hid away like a hermit writing this book. I would also like to thank my lovely sister Darla Shelley and my best friend Jeffrey Bell for their kind edits and support through many early drafts of this book. Thanks also to my dear friends Randi Barshack, Bob Bogard, Steven Freedman, Melisa Milkie, Keith Pascale, Aileen Schulte, Ingrid Seyer-Ochi, Erica Sharkansky, and Dan Shelley for their many great ideas and words of encouragement over the years.

Finally, profound thanks to my agent, Margaret Gee, for her extraordinary efforts in the worst publishing market ever, and also to my editor, Shana Drehs, for helping to bring a coherent order and vision to this project.

Introduction

Who Should You Have Sex With?

This is a bold and daring question. It speaks to the increased freedom we enjoy sexually and the new decisions and responsibilities that come with this freedom.

A few decades ago the question of "who should you have sex with" was not relevant to most men and women, because they married young and stayed married for most of their lives. But times have changed. People marry later than they used to, and at least half divorce at some point in their lives. We're spending longer and longer stretches of our lives single and on the market for both sex and romance.

The Internet has also dramatically changed our relationships and sex lives. Over fifty million men and women use the Internet to find dates, sex, and romance each year. In my studies of online daters, I found that about *half* say they are looking for a "sexually passionate" romance and want to have a "great sex life" with their future partner.

The other half place less importance on sexual passion, but they assign a higher priority to romantic love and relationship trust and stability. But sex (or ambivalence about sex) still plays a big role in their dating lives. Many of them are also curious about who would make the best bedroom partner and debate whether or not (and when) to take things to a sexual level. They also worry about ending up with a partner who wants *more* sex (or kinkier sex) than they are interested in.

Questions about sex are playing a bigger role in the lives of couples as well. People expect more out of their marriages than ever before. Couples are less likely to settle for sexual boredom and the loss of sexual chemistry than they used to. For better or for worse, the expectations we bring to our sex lives have shot way up. So, at some point, most couples will ask if the person in their bed is the person they want to be making love to for the rest of their lives.

How Do I Know This?

I have spent the last decade looking over America's shoulder, studying how men and women look for love, sex, and relationships online. I helped design matching systems for the two largest online dating websites: Match.com and Yahoo! I created interactive online tests about physical attraction, personality types, love styles, and sexual interests, and I gathered data on the preferences and passions of more than thirty million men and women who have taken one or more of my tests.

I've seen a lot on my journey through the Internet dating world. As a clinical psychologist and researcher by training, it's in my nature to look for themes and trends and to try to make sense of what I observe. It won't surprise you to learn that a lot of the activity I observed online and a lot of the exchanges and frustrations people reported had to do with sex. Sex plays a big role in online dating. There's a lot of talk about sex; there are a lot of people having sex.

Yet I've come to believe there are some very important questions about sex and relationships that no one is asking.

What Questions Should We Be Asking?

Most people fall into one of two extremes when it comes to talking about sex: they either refuse to talk about sex directly, or they talk about sex too soon or too explicitly. Since I've written a whole book about sex, I obviously favor talking about it. Most of us have inherited our society's conflicted attitude toward sex. I've personally spent large chunks of my life cycling between obsession and avoidance when it comes to sex. Neither is a healthy or happy place to be. So I'm a big advocate for knowing and understanding your sexual self and being able to talk about your interests and desires with your partner or potential partner.

Still, even people who are comfortable talking about sex tend to have a relatively narrow set of topics they discuss. On the rare occasion that people talk about sexual compatibility, they usually focus on how often they like to have sex. Some may even talk about their favorite sexual activities or positions. But these issues only cover part of what it means to be sexually compatible.

So, in this book, I'm going to ask you to take a big step back and ask a more fundamental question: who should you have sex with? We'll look at the type of connection and type of lover you need in order to have a truly great sex life. This question is obviously relevant to single men and women who are looking for a lover or a long-term partner. But I think that married men and women can learn something from asking this question as well. If you're not 100 percent happy with your sex life, exploring the type of lover you find most appealing as well as the qualities you bring to the bedroom can help you understand what the two of you as a couple can do to reignite or realign your sexual chemistry.

The difference between the best sexual connection you've ever had and the worst probably had little to do with the frequency or mechanics of sex. It probably had everything to do with *how* you had sex. You and your favorite lover probably both approached sex in a similar way—as wholesome and fun or maybe as nasty and naughty. You probably both liked having sex at a similar pace—slow and sensual or fast and intense. Chances are, one of you liked to take charge, while the other enjoyed surrendering and losing control.

So in order to know who you should have sex with, we need to expand our sexual vocabulary and explore the factors that go into creating initial sexual chemistry as well as long-term sexual compatibility. We need to understand how you approach sex and the type of lover who best fits your sexual style.

What Will This Book Teach You?

By the end of this book, you'll understand your own sexual desires in a way that you may have never thought possible. You'll also gain expertise in reading the secret desires of your current (or future) partner. I'll teach you the ingredients that go into creating great sexual chemistry and how to spot these qualities in a partner. For those of you already in a relationship, I'll show you how to reignite your sexual spark by exploring your and your partner's sexual fantasies and trying out new sexual roles.

We'll learn from the experiences of real men and women like you. This book brings together the results of over one hundred separate studies with over six million men and women from ages eighteen to eighty that I conducted with a multidisciplinary team of psychologists, sociologists, health educators, and statisticians. It's this research and the interactive exercises I developed based on this research that set this book apart from most books about sex that focus on opinions and advice. I'm not against opinions; I have lots of them. But in this book, I try to stay as close as I can to the research data. The result is a story that is a thousand times more interesting, complex, and surprising than any sexy magazine article or self-help book could offer.

I divided the book into four parts. Parts 1 and 3 focus on what I've learned from my studies of millions of men and women. The chapters in these sections map out a framework for understanding the components of sexual compatibility and sexual chemistry. You'll have a chance to explore your own tastes and preferences and the types of qualities you find most appealing in a lover.

I organized the parts of the book so that we can alternate between insights and application. Part 2 focuses on the applications and implications of the information you'll learn in Part 1. Similarly, Part 4 applies the insights from Part 3. Every chapter includes interactive exercises, based on my online tests, and a chance to compare your choices to those of other men or women like you. Even though the book is based on research, I've tried to make it as fun as possible. Sex is supposed to be fun, right?! To give you a better idea of what lies ahead, let's look at the goals of each part of the book.

Part 1: What Are the Basics of a Satisfying and Lasting Sexual Connection?

In Part 1, we'll look at the first two cornerstones of sexual compatibility: (1) similar sex drives and (2) similar interests in sexual variety and adventurousness.

Each chapter in Part 1 focuses on a key question you should ask yourself and your sexual partner (or future partner) in order to gauge whether you could have a potentially lasting and satisfying sexual connection. I've translated my popular online tests about sexual variety and kinky tastes into exercises to help you identify your unique preferences and desires. You'll also be able to compare your preferences with those of millions of men and women like you.

Part 2: How Can You Find (or Create) Sexual Compatibility?

Part 2 offers practical advice on how to find and create compatibility in sex drives and sexual adventurousness.

For those of you who wonder if there is a way to spot potentially compatible partners *before* you ask them out on a date, I share (in Chapter 3) new research on the link between external traits and people's inner sexual desires. We'll see how qualities such as shyness, intelligence, dependability, and niceness may offer clues to a potential date's sex drive and sexual adventurousness. You can't always judge a book by its cover. But knowing the traits to look for may help you decide where to invest your dating energies.

For readers already in a relationship, Chapter 4 looks at ways to maintain your sexual compatibility over time and offers practical advice on dealing with different sex drives, making monogamy work, and dealing with sexual boredom. There are exercises to help you talk with your partner about your sexual interests, fears, and insecurities.

Part 3: Secrets of Sexual Chemistry

Sexual chemistry is different from sexual compatibility. Chemistry is something you create in the moment as part of your sexual connection with someone. You can see chemistry at work (or its absence) in a single sexual encounter or re-created again and again throughout a relationship.

In Part 3, we'll move beyond the basics of sexual compatibility and look at the deeper challenges involved in finding (or creating) good sexual chemistry. We will see how the basic ingredients of sexual chemistry come together in a single encounter and how (if you're lucky) you can find a partner who can re-create this formula again and again over the long haul.

I'll ask you to think about the best sexual connections you've ever had and the specific combination of factors that made your best sex so great. We'll look at each of the facets of sexual chemistry in depth. Using fun exercises, we'll explore (1) if you enjoy the lighter or darker side of sex, (2) if being dominant or submissive turns you on, and (3) if you like sex that is fast and intense or slow and gentle. You'll learn about your own personal recipe for great sex and which combination of ingredients works best for you.

Part 3 also explores the complexities and mysteries that surround the distinction between our public selves and our private sexual selves. One of the surprising things about dating (which no one prepares you for) is that the person you meet and have dinner with is not always the same person you meet when the lights go off in your bedroom. The public personality you are initially drawn to may be nothing like the sexual personality that comes out when you get naked.

To my knowledge, this is the first book to map out a framework for understanding sexual personalities and how they overlap or are distinct from other parts of your personality. We'll look at how the three facets of sexual chemistry (emotional tone, power, and activity) combine to create eight *sexual personas* (with names like Mr./Ms. Dominant, Mr./Ms. Playful, and Mr./Ms. Passion).

We'll see how these different styles and approaches to sex express themselves in your inner sex life and fantasies and in your interpersonal sex life and relationships. In Part 3, I share for the first time the results of a national study on men's and women's favorite sexual fantasies. I describe the most popular sexual characters, settings, and activities. I also present a framework for understanding what your fantasies say about your sexual desires and the sexual fears and inhibitions your fantasies try to overcome.

Part 4: Improving Your Sexual Chemistry

Part 4 looks at ways to transform the quality of your sex life by improving the sexual chemistry you share with your partner. For single folks, this starts with finding a partner with a sexual persona that meshes with your own. I'll show you how to watch for clues in people's behavior and their public personality that can help you predict their sexual style. We'll look at why it's so important to recognize, talk about, and celebrate the sexual complexities in you and your potential partner.

For readers already in a relationship, we'll look at how sexual personas can change over time and what happens when two people's sexual styles drift apart or pull in opposite directions. Fortunately, there are several things you can do to reignite your sexual spark and realign your sexual chemistry. Through interactive exercises, you'll learn how to be a better lover by finding the exact combination of emotion, power, and intensity that will turn your partner on.

Finally, we'll explore how to use sexual role-play to expand your sexual style and try out new ways of relating to each other sexually. I'll share new research on the most popular role-play scenarios among both women and men. Of all the tools and techniques in this book, I believe talking about your sexual fantasies with your partner and then acting them out through role-play have the biggest potential to transform your sex life and reignite your sexual spark.

Are You Ready for the Journey?

You are starting the book where I'm ending it, since I wrote this introduction last. Writing this book has been quite a journey. It was a bigger investment of time, energy, and money than I ever could have imagined. As with so many things in life, it probably worked out for the best that I had no idea what I was getting into when I started it.

By reading the book, you've embarked on a journey as well. You've decided to invest time, money, and energy in yourself and your current or future relationship. You may have no idea what you're getting into. I expect the topics and exercises in this book will open doors that lead to some exciting places, but they may also open doors to some difficult or uncomfortable places.

I believe this journey of sexual self-discovery is worth the investment. In fact, I can think of no other personal cause that is more worthy, more misunderstood, more neglected, more desperately needed, and ultimately more rewarding.

PART 1

What Are the Basics of a Satisfying and Lasting Sexual Connection?

Chapter 1

Sex Drive

How Often Do You Want Sex?

Why We Want Sex

What Motivates Us to Have Sex?

Before we can explore *who* you should have sex with, we need to start by asking, Why do you want to have sex in the first place? When I give lectures and raise this question, someone in the audience usually jokes that if I have to ask, I don't get out enough. That's probably true, and I'm the first to admit it. So I usually ask my younger and worldlier audience to refresh my memory: Why do we think about sex so much and want to have it so often?

"To have babies" is a popular response.

I agree. Sex is essential to procreation. Still, I point out that even if you have three kids (a big family today), these three conceptions will account for an extremely small proportion of your sexual experiences. If you take into account that at least half of all pregnancies are unintentional, then sex with the *goal* of reproduction is especially rare.

With some further prompting, people usually offer the following reasons for why we want sex: Sex feels good. It's pleasurable. It keeps relationships together. It's an escape from the real world.

Within these top-of-mind answers are three core psychological motivations for sex. Specifically, they refer to three kinds of reinforcement.

First and most obviously, sex is a reward or positive reinforcement. Even thinking about sex is arousing and can put a mischievous smile on your face. And real sex with a partner is not only physically pleasurable, but it also offers emotional and psychological rewards: feeling loved, wanted, valued, and so forth. Sex is also rewarding to you as a couple, since it reinforces and strengthens your bond with each other.

Of course, whether you are single or in a relationship, there will be times when you put a lot of effort into having sex, albeit with little or no success. In other words, you can't always count on that reward. I personally have been shot down and ignored in cities around the world. There have also been times (due to no fault of my own, of course) when sex has not been especially enjoyable. Still, I have never stopped wanting sex. Chances are you haven't given up on it either. Why?

One explanation is that the search for good sex is itself reinforcing. Sure, the destination is great, but the journey can be fun too. Researchers who study brain functioning in other animals have found that the parts of the brain that prompt animals to seek out sex also promote other so-called seeking behaviors, such as foraging, hunting, and exploring new territory.[1] Their brains release dopamine and other stimulating chemicals that make them enjoy seeking out and exploring their environment. So perhaps our brains reward us along the way as well when we seek out sex.

How Does Failure and Only Periodic Success Get Us Hooked on Sex?

Another reason we keep wanting sex, despite endless delays and frustrations, is that sex is a powerful *intermittent reinforcement*. If you give a mouse a reward (like a pellet of food) every time he pushes a button, he will keep pushing the button as long as you give him the reward. But if you stop rewarding him, he'll quickly figure out that the jig is up and stop pushing the button. If, however, you give the reward at random (or intermittent) intervals, then he will keep pushing the button long after you've left the room. Because the rewards come sporadically, the little mouse has no way of knowing when to stop trying.

As this mouse and anyone who's played slot machines at a casino will tell you, rewards that come in the form of intermittent reinforcement are the most difficult to walk away from. As long as you win an occasional jackpot on those penny slot machines, you can be stuck in that casino for days.

Oddly enough, sex is like that too. It's the failures and frustrations we encounter in our sex lives that keep us most committed to sex over the long term. The superstud who never encounters rejection is caught off guard and easily discouraged when his looks start to fade and he's no longer the hottest ticket in town. Meanwhile, the rest of us keep on dating or keep making efforts to keep the spark alive in our relationship, not because we expect to always succeed, but because of the great times we've had before and the chance that it can happen again.

How Is Sex a Negative Reinforcement?

The third motivating force behind our desire for sex comes in the form of *negative reinforcement*. If you're a smarty-pants who enjoys correcting other people, be sure to take notes here. I frequently hear people, even experts who should know better, mistakenly use the term *negative reinforcement* as a fancy way of saying *punishment*. Negative reinforcement is a reward, *not* a punishment. It encourages a behavior (or a desire) by removing a negative state. While positive reinforcement moves you from a neutral state to a more pleasurable one, negative reinforcement moves you from an unpleasant state back to a neutral state or better.

Food is a good example of negative reinforcement. Delicious food is obviously a positive reinforcement, but even mediocre food can be a reinforcement if you're hungry. Hunger is an unpleasant state, and food functions to remove our hunger pains.

If you're in a negative state, such as being bored or depressed, sex can be energizing, invigorating, and make you feel young. If you are feeling anxious and agitated about work or other stressors in your life, sex can be a good distraction, soothe your nerves, and relax you.

People use sex in the same way they use music to help regulate their moods. Sometimes music can boost your energy level, like when you're working out at the gym. At other times, we look to music to calm us.

Sex also relieves unhappiness. It can reduce feelings of loneliness (even if only temporarily). Sex also helps iron over tensions in a relationship; thus, the joy of make-up sex.

I'm not a big fan of the term *horny*. However, to the extent that this refers to an unpleasant state of excessive sexual desire, sex can function as a negative reinforcement by relieving horniness as well.

To sum up, we want to find someone who is worth sleeping with because sex is both pleasurable and soothing. It minimizes our bad emotional states and increases positive feelings. It's a big reward. Even though we can't always get sex when we want it—and when we get it, we don't always find it satisfying—we still keep pursuing it because we are hooked on the intermittent rewards that we've encountered in the past. Ironically, it's the challenge we face in getting and enjoying sex that keeps us hooked on sex most of our lives.

For all these reasons, the vast majority of men and women want to have sex (at least occasionally). As we explore who you should have sex with, the question often turns to how much sex you want and how much sex your potential partner wants. Let's look at one approach to sorting this out.

Levels of Sex Drive

Is Sex Really a Drive?

Your *sex drive* corresponds to the total amount of time and energy you put into thinking about sex, pursuing sex, and having sex—both solo sex and partner sex.

I'm not a big fan of the term *sex drive*. I don't believe we are *driven* to have sex. I don't believe sex is a biological imperative. Many of us certainly want sex a great deal (and often), but it's not a biological need or necessity, like eating or drinking. We humans *want* a lot of things: delicious food, nice clothes, fast cars, etc. We're also *passionate* about a lot of issues and activities: gardening, fishing, wine tasting, video game playing, etc. Yet no one suggests that women have an instinctual "shoe drive" or that men have biologically driven "sports passions."

However, old habits die hard. For almost two decades, I've used the term *sex drive* to refer to how often people think about sex and want to have sex. And frankly, I'm too stuck in my ways to change my lexicon. So I'm going to take the easy way out and continue to use the term *sex drive* but still do my best to avoid implying that sex is driven by some biological bogeyman who pulls our puppet strings.

Is Your Sex Drive High or Low: The Shortcut Answer to This Question

To identify the level of your sex drive, you can either take the shortcut approach or a more thorough approach. The shortcut is mapped out in Exercise 1 (for women) and Exercise 2 (for men) and focuses on three questions:

- How often do you think about sex?
- When you are single, how often do you masturbate?
- When you are in a relationship, how often do you like to have sex?

If you have fast and straightforward answers to these questions, jump ahead to the exercise. For those of you interested in a more thorough review, let's tackle each of these arenas separately.

How Often Do You Think about Sex?

The first sexual arena—our internal mental and fantasy world—is the most difficult for us to capture and quantify. It's hard to ever be fully aware of what we're thinking about or imaging. They call the flow of cognitions in our mind the stream of consciousness, but it's really more like a river, with dozens of tributaries of ideas, plans, memories, and daydreams flowing in and out of our awareness at any given moment.

How much of this cognition is sexual? I think it's close to impossible to nail down. But as a start, think about the last time you:

- remembered a previous sexual experience;
- undressed someone with your eyes;
- imagined what it would be like to have sex with one of your friends, co-workers, or someone famous;
- daydreamed or fantasized about a sexual experience you'd like to have;
- anticipated the possibility of having sex tonight, tomorrow, or next week.

Since sex is just one of many things your mind can be interested in and passionate about, try to think about how much you think about sex compared to other parts of your life. Imagine your brain is like a radio station. How much airtime is dedicated to your sexual interests or daydreams? How does this compare with the airtime you give to thinking about your friends, family, pets, favorite sports team, favorite television shows, etc.? Is sex a big part of your airtime programming or just an occasional special report or emergency bulletin?

People with high sex drives think about sex and sexual possibilities at least once a day and often several times a day. People with moderate sex drives know they think about sex, but they have a harder time specifying what they think about and whether it is every day or every few days. People with low sex drives rarely think about sex or have a specific sexual fantasy or daydream. They tend to give much more mental airtime to other interests and passions.

How Often Do You Masturbate?

The second sexual arena centers on the ways you actively explore your sexuality when you're alone. Time spent exploring a sexual fantasy, reading erotica, looking at porn, or surfing the Internet for sexual content all fall into this category.

Most single men and women (and a significant number of partnered men and women) say they masturbate on a regular basis. It turns out that there are several varieties of and motivations for masturbation. The most common form is *masturbation as a substitute for sex*. It's something you do to burn off sexual energy because you lack a sexual partner or your regular partner is out of town or otherwise unavailable.

The second most common form is *masturbation as a supplement for partner sex*. Here, masturbation is simply an additional sexual outlet for individuals who have a lot of sexual energy and not enough opportunities to have sex with their partner.

The final variety can best be described as *solo sex*. This kind of masturbation lets you explore desires and fantasies that you prefer not to talk about or act out with a partner. Solo sex can give you the opportunity to stimulate yourself exactly the way you like, at the pace you like, and for as long as you like. For some men and women, solo sex is also a way to explore private fantasies that are immensely pleasurable but also a source of confusion, guilt, or shame. We'll take a closer look at these sorts of masturbation fantasies in Chapter 9.

As a rule, people with high sex drives enjoy all three forms of masturbation on a regular basis. When they're single, they masturbate almost daily, and even when they are in a relationship, they still masturbate periodically to let off steam or explore their secret desires or fantasies. Men and women with moderate sex drives tend to approach masturbation as an occasional necessity and substitute for "real sex." People with low sex drives rarely masturbate and are the least likely to enjoy solo sex.

How Often Do You Want to Have Sex with Your Partner?

The third arena involves the ways you express your sexual desire with others. If you are in a relationship, this includes how often and how long you have sex with your partner. If you are single, this includes the frequency and duration of your sexual connections while dating or with sex buddies or other sexual outlets. My definition of sex includes making out, all three "bases," and pretty much any erotic or arousing play.

As you know, life and relationships have a way of frustrating our desires. As we'll examine throughout this book, there are many potential barriers to finding a partner and finding a sexually compatible partner. Put another way, you can't always get what you want, especially if what you want is sex.

So another important gauge of sexual desire is how often you would *like* to have sex with a partner. If you could orchestrate your life exactly the way you wanted, would you have sex every day, every few days, every week, every couple of weeks, or just every full moon?

Figure 1 outlines how men and women answer this question.[2] About one in five men want to have sex every day. Slightly fewer women want sex on a daily basis. The distribution of men and women across the other groups is very similar. About one in three men and women want to have sex a few times a week; another one in three want

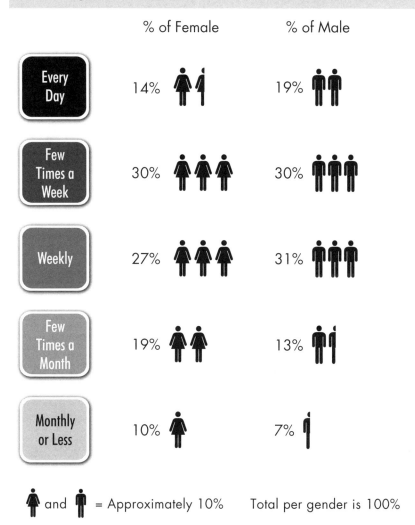

Figure 1: How Often Do You Like to Have Sex?

to have sex about once a week. Finally, about one in three women and one in five men want to have sex a few times a month or less.

So, despite gender stereotypes that suggest all men are sex maniacs while most women are frigid, my research points to a wide range of sexual desires among both men and women. Slightly more men than women want daily sex, and somewhat more women fall

Exercise 1: Women's Sex Drive

How often do you have a

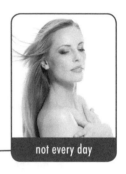

not every day

When single, how often do you masturbate?

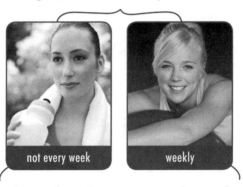

not every week — weekly

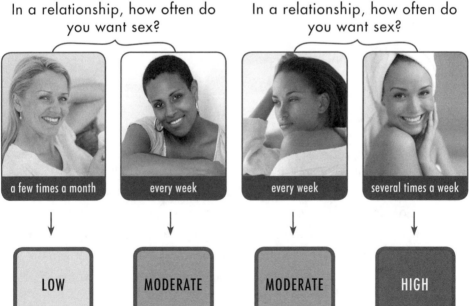

In a relationship, how often do you want sex?   In a relationship, how often do you want sex?

a few times a month   every week   every week   several times a week

LOW   MODERATE   MODERATE   HIGH

sexual daydream or fantasy?

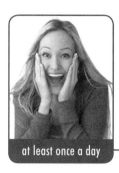

at least once a day

When single, how often do you masturbate?

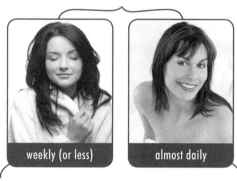

weekly (or less) almost daily

In a relationship, how often do you want sex?

In a relationship, how often do you want sex?

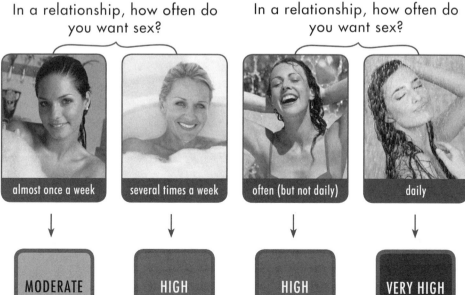

almost once a week several times a week often (but not daily) daily

MODERATE HIGH HIGH VERY HIGH

Exercise 2: Men's Sex Drive

How often do you have a

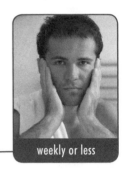

weekly or less

When single, how often do you masturbate?

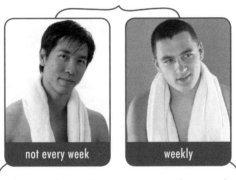

not every week   weekly

In a relationship, how often do you want sex?   In a relationship, how often do you want sex?

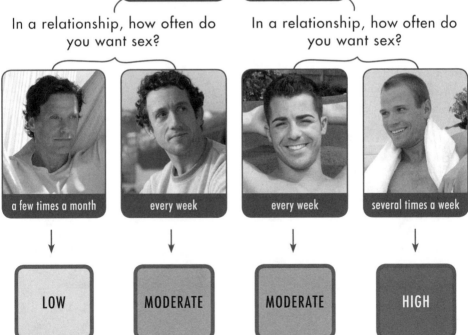

a few times a month   every week   every week   several times a week

LOW   MODERATE   MODERATE   HIGH

sexual daydream or fantasy?

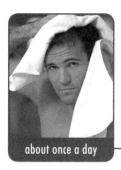

When single, how often do you masturbate?

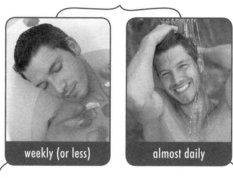

In a relationship, how often do you want sex?

In a relationship, how often do you want sex?

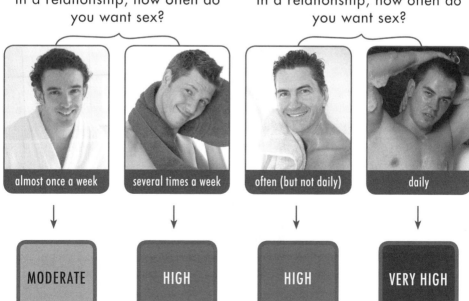

at the other extreme of wanting sex infrequently. For the most part, though, there are similar clusters of men and women at each of the preference levels.

Do You Have a High Sex Drive?

If you haven't already, take a moment to complete either Exercise 1 or 2. You can use your insights from the previous three sections to guide where you branch off at each of the three decision points. Your choices should lead you to one of four sex drive categories: low, moderate, high, or very high.

Most people expect they will end up in one of the high sex drive categories. So if the exercise sorted you into either the low or moderate category, you may be surprised or disappointed.

In surveys, we've asked hundreds of thousands of people: "Do you have a *high* sex drive?"[3] Consistently, in survey after survey, the majority of men *and* women say yes.

I think people's competitive nature takes over when they hear this question, and they equate *high* with good and *low* with bad or deficient. A lot of men and women assume that a normal person has a high sex drive. But the research suggests otherwise. Most men and women do not think about sex, masturbate, or have sex every day.

How Many Men and Women Fall into Each Category?

Let's take a brief look at each of the four sex drive levels. In Figure 2, I've listed the proportion of men and women who fit into each of the categories.

Figure 2: Levels of Sex Drive among Women and Men

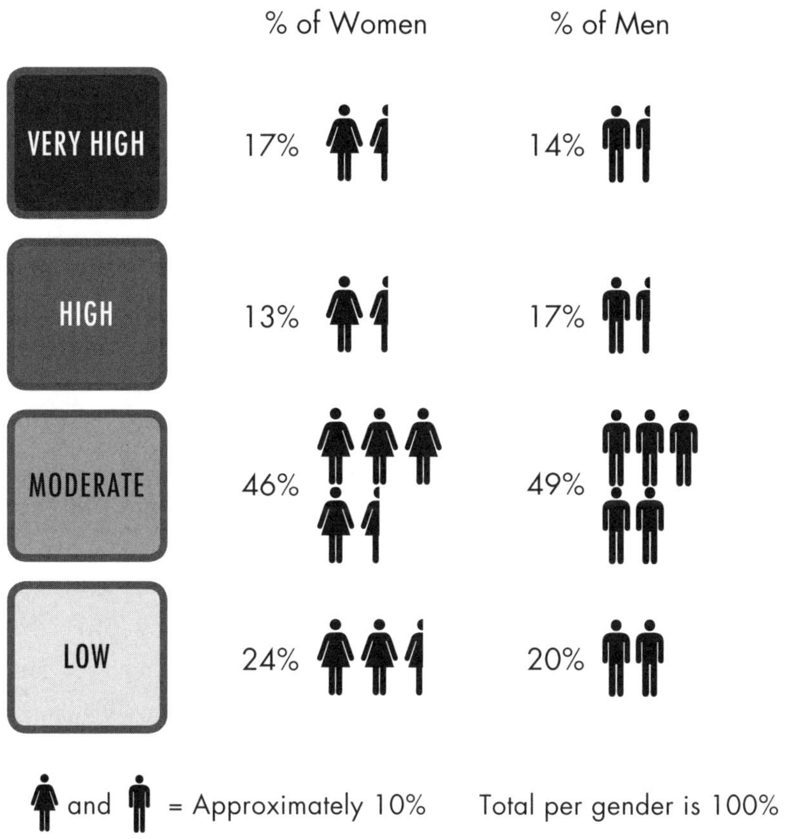

	% of Women	% of Men
VERY HIGH	17%	14%
HIGH	13%	17%
MODERATE	46%	49%
LOW	24%	20%

👩 and 👨 = Approximately 10%   Total per gender is 100%

Individuals with *very high* sex drives think about sex and want some outlet for their desire every single day. They daydream or fantasize about sex at least once a day, masturbate every day (when they are single), and want to have sex every day (when they are in a relationship).

Obviously, sex plays an important and prominent role in their lives. Being a very sexual person is part of how they see themselves. Sex usually serves many functions in their lives. It's fun and pleasurable, but it also serves as an escape from stress and a way to soothe tensions.

They tend to want sex early in a relationship and believe a good sex life is essential to making a long-term relationship work. In fact, they typically have little patience for staying in a relationship if the passion dies.

About one in seven adults fit the criteria for very high sex drive. This is consistent across men and women. As you'll recall, slightly more men than women want to have sex every day. However, once you take into account the frequency of thinking about sex and the frequency of masturbation, there's no gender difference in the proportion who occupy this highest sex drive tier.

Individuals with a *high* sex drive also think about sex at least once a day. However, they are a bit more flexible about how often they need to express their desire and about the outlet for their desire. They tend to masturbate about once a week when they are single and prefer to have sex a few times a week when in a relationship.

About one in seven men and women fall in this category. This breakout also remains fairly consistent across age groups. However, the proportion of men with high sex drives peaks at about age thirty, while the proportion peaks among women at about age forty.

In the framework I've outlined, there are several routes to having a *moderate* sex drive. People with moderate sex drives tend to masturbate at least occasionally when they are single and want to have sex in a relationship about once a week. Regular sex for pleasure or release is an important part of this person's life. However, it's not a prominent or essential feature in his or her day-to-day life. Approximately half of all adults fall in the moderate drive category as it is defined here.

On the other end of the continuum are people with a *low* overall interest in sex. They do not think about sex every day and can go a week or more without either masturbating or having sex with their partner. This does not mean that they dislike sex. In most cases, they simply have other life passions (like work, family, exercise, cooking, gardening, etc.) that occupy their thoughts and energy. About one in five men and one in three women fall in the low sex drive category.

Do You Want a Partner with a High or Low Sex Drive?

You can also use the charts in Exercise 1 or 2 to consider what level of sex drive you would want your ideal partner to have. Pick the exercise with photos of the gender you're attracted to and ask yourself at each of the branches: Do you want a partner who fantasizes about sex every day or less often? If you were out of town for a week, would you want a partner who would need to masturbate every day, once, or not at all? Do you want a partner who will want to have sex every day, every few days, weekly, or less?

When I asked single men and women these questions, the vast majority said they were looking for a partner whose sex drive is similar to their own. In fact, 92 percent of *women* say they want a partner who thinks about sex and wants to have sex exactly as often as they do.

Interestingly, one in four men say they want a partner who wants sex *more often* than they do. I am not sure what this finding means, although it pops up again and again in my research. Several men have explained that having a partner who wants sex more often than you do increases the odds that you will at least get to have sex whenever *you* want to. If she's always in the mood, I guess they figure they'll never get turned down. This may sound good in the abstract, but as we'll see in Part 2, having different sex drives is usually less than ideal for both parties, even if you're the one getting sex as often as you'd like.

Is There a Downside to Having a Partner with a High Sex Drive?

When you look at the sexual histories of men and women with high sex drives, several things stand out. First, as you'd expect, people with high or very high sex drives are much more sexually experienced than people with low or moderate drives. So if you're hoping to find a partner with a high sex drive who's been sexually pure and saving herself (or himself) for you, you can forget it.

People with high sex drives tend to bring a fair amount of sexual baggage or a lot of good practice, depending on how you look at it. Compared to individuals with low or moderate sex drives, men and women with high or very high sex drives are *twice* as likely to report having had twenty or more sexual partners and *twice* as likely to recall having several one-night stands. They are also *twice* as likely to say they have made a decision in a moment of sexual passion that they later regretted.

In my research, compared to those with low or moderate sex drives, men and women with high or very high sex drives were also *twice* as likely to say they had cheated on their partner while in a monogamous relationship. The risk of infidelity appears to be especially pronounced for individuals in the *very high* sex drive category. About two in five men (39 percent) and one in five women (21 percent) with very high sex drives say they have "sexually strayed while in a committed relationship."

Therefore, the upside of having a partner with a high sex drive is that they want a lot of sex, and you will likely get to have sex whenever you want it. The downside is that they want a lot of sex and may be more likely to seek it outside of your relationship than would a partner with a lower sex drive.

Who Is Attracted to Men and Women with Low Sex Drives?

The vast majority of men and women with low sex drives say they want a partner who also has a low sex drive. So individuals with low sex drives are certainly desirable and sought-after partners, especially by other men and women with low drives.

With that said, there is definitely a stigma attached to men who are not sexually active. The vast majority of women (80 percent) say they are *not* interested in dating a man who is sexually chaste or who has never had sexual intercourse.

Men are somewhat more accepting of meeting a partner who is still a virgin. About half (46 percent) are open to dating a partner who is a virgin, and one in ten (12 percent) say a woman who has saved her virginity is extremely appealing.

If you're looking for a sexually chaste man or woman, keep in mind that he or she is very likely to fall in the low sex drive category. In my studies, over half of all virgins in their twenties and thirties, as well as the iconic forty-year-old virgins, report rarely thinking about or fantasizing about sex. They also tend to masturbate less often than their nonchaste peers.

It's unclear whether they've remained virgins because they have little interest in sex or whether they intentionally suppress sexual thoughts and masturbation in order to maintain their virginity. Regardless, if you meet a sexual late bloomer, keep in mind that he or she is probably "shut down" sexually and may not ever be a very sexual person.

Who Is Most and Least Worried about Sexual Performance and Infidelity?

Another interesting thing about men and women with low sex drives is their mild indifference to sexual problems and infidelity. Most men and women say they worry about pleasing their partner sexually. In fact, two out of three people with very high sex drives say they get upset if they cannot perform sexually or satisfy their partner. People with low sex drives tend to be much less concerned about sexual performance; only one in four (23 percent) say they would be upset if they couldn't satisfy their partner sexually.

Although most people want a partner who is sexually faithful, the people *most* worried about infidelity are those with very high sex drives. It's probably not a coincidence that the men and women with high sex drives who are the most likely to have been unfaithful in past relationships are also the most worried about having a partner who will cheat on them in the future. While the vast majority of men and women with high (or very high) sex drives (82 percent) say it is *very* important to have a partner who is sexually faithful, only half of those with low sexual drives (52 percent) say this is very important. This doesn't mean that people with low sex drives tend to accept infidelity, but it does mean that they are less concerned about it or see it as a deal breaker.

What Is Too Much or Too Little?

One of the reasons I dislike the sex drive lingo is because it's easy to phrase things in a way that implies that people with low sex drives are deficient in some way or that people with high sex drives are excessive or obsessive in their fondness for sex. It is easy to fall into the trap, like Goldilocks, of comparing groups of people like bowls of porridge and finding one to be too hot or too cold and one just right. There is no *right* level of sexual desire. In my opinion, experts who say they know the right level or insist everyone conform to some abstract ideal deserve to be mauled by bears like Goldilocks.

Pop psychology, for example, promotes a myth that only sexually passionate couples can be happy. A sexual connection is only one of the potential building blocks for a romantic relationship. Some couples place more importance on shared goals, friendship, or raising a family than on sexual compatibility. Similarly, they may prefer affection and emotional intimacy over physical intimacy. If these couples are happy together, who's to say their relationship is somehow deficient?

In fact, who's to say that one has to have a partner or be sexually active in order to enjoy a productive and rewarding life? People with low sex drives are more likely than their peers to say they are okay with not having a romantic partner.

One can certainly find numerous role models in history and literature who channeled their time and energy into creative, scholarly, or humanitarian pursuits rather than a romantic or sexual life. Think of the naturalist and author Henry David Thoreau or the humanitarian accomplishments of Eleanor Roosevelt or Mother Teresa. The brilliant religious scholar and bestselling author Karen Armstrong is a modern-day example of someone who created a rewarding and fulfilling life while being celibate.

If people with low sex drives are portrayed as being deficient or lacking some important psychological "fuel," people with high sex drives are often portrayed as having excessive urges and desires. There's certainly a point where too much time and energy focused on sex can become destructive. People who suffer from sexual obsessions and compulsions experience sex as an addiction that interferes with their ability to live and enjoy their lives. But the vast majority of men and women with very high sex drives are not obsessed with sex; they simply find it more interesting and enjoyable than most people.

Some people simply bring more energy, emotional intensity, and dedication to their interests than others. We all know people who bring intense passion to their careers. I know I used to—before I got middle-aged and lazy. We've all seen amateur and professional athletes push themselves to obscene lengths for sports. Artists are also prone to manic bursts of dancing, painting, or other creative outbursts. Even hobbies tend to inspire a level of dedication and excitement that nondevotees find hard to understand. As humor columnist Dave Barry expressed it, "There is a very fine line between a 'hobby' and 'mental illness.'"

Keep in mind that the right level of sexual desire for you will probably change over the course of your life. Your sex drive is not a fixed quantity. The frequency with which you think about sex or want to have sex will change as you age and depending on your life circumstances. You may go through periods when you are very interested in sex and then through periods when you are not. The same applies to anyone you choose to have sex with.

So I hope you can accept and feel good about your sex drive—whatever its level. I also hope you can understand and appreciate your partner's sex drive as well, even if it is higher or lower than your own. As we'll see in Part 2, there are a number of things you can do as a couple to cope with different sexual desires. But these efforts have to start with a loving acceptance of yourself and each other for who you are and what you bring sexually to your relationship. There are no good or bad levels of sexual desire, no right or wrong levels. You can find happy and unhappy people at every level.

Chapter 2

Sexual Variety

How Sexually Adventurous Are You?

Exploring Sexual Variety

What Is Your Favorite Kind of Sex?

Now that we've covered how often you like to have sex, we can turn to the juicy details and look at what you like to do sexually. Let's start by mapping out your sexual favorites. Take a moment and think about your answer to each of these questions:

- *What* are your favorite sexual activities?
- *Where* do you like to have sex?
- *When* are you most in the mood for sex?
- *How* do you like sex to unfold? Do you have a preferred sequence for what happens first and last?

Let's assume you could have sex exactly this way and do exactly what you like, when, where, and how you like it. If you could experience this exact scenario every time you had sex, would you be interested in having sex this way, without variation, for the next year?

Your answer to this last question points to the core challenge in finding your ideal sexually compatible partner. If you said, "Yes, please, I would love to have sex this way for a full year," then the challenge is finding a partner who enjoys the same sexual menu as you do.

If you said, "No, I'd eventually get bored doing the exact same thing," then you face an extra challenge. You have to find a partner who likes to mix things up sexually in the same way you do. In this chapter, we're going to explore three kinds of sexual variety: variations in sexual activities, the role of sexual creativity, and your openness to exploring kinky sex.

If I Like My Sexual Routine, Do I Still Need Variety?

Even if you answered, "Yes, please," to having your favorite sexual routine over and over again, I'm still going to encourage you to find some areas where you might be open to sexual variety. But you may ask, If I'm happy with my sexual routine, why should I mess with a good thing?

I don't have anything against sexual routines, especially if they are satisfying to both partners. Sometimes sexual routines can be comforting sexual rituals. They have a predictable beginning, middle, and end. They are comforting in part because you know what's going to happen. You can let yourself go and enjoy the carefree flow of sexual sensations.

Still, even the best sexual routine can become predictable and lackluster over time. So if you're going to keep the sexual spark alive in your relationship, you need to be able to mix things up occasionally. This chapter can help you (and your partner) identify the types of sexual variety you'd be open to and what you can do to expand your repertoire of sexual rituals.

How Adventurous Are You with Food?

There are three categories of sexual variety. Yes, there are varieties of variety. I never said this was going to be easy!

To introduce you to each of these dimensions, I want you to think about how you approach food and your openness to experimenting with different culinary experiences. Although this may seem like a bit of a detour, there's a method to my madness, so try to just go with it.

First question: How often do you like to try new or different kinds of food?

People tend to fall on a continuum from those with very limited and routine diets to those who are constantly trying new kinds of food. I definitely fall more toward the routine end of the continuum. I have had peanut butter on toast for breakfast every morning for the past twenty years and loved it every single time.

Even if you're not that rigid, you probably have some consistency in your menus from week to week. You probably pick up a similar set of items each time you go to the grocery store.

Is there an average cuisine that most people prefer? That may have been the case fifty years ago. In fact, a 1954 poll found that the majority of Americans said their favorite or ideal meal consisted of a fruit cup, vegetable soup, a steak, French fries, peas, and apple pie a la mode.[4] Today, I doubt anyone would choose to eat this exact menu. Fruit cups are so fifty years ago!

Still, there is certainly a subgroup of Americans who prefer meat and potatoes over foreign or exotic foods. Some people love trying new restaurants and are curious to sample the latest cuisines. The hot new restaurant in my neighborhood, for example, serves only raw and uncooked food. They have a line of people waiting to get in every night, but most of my friends refuse to go with me to such an allegedly bizarre establishment.

Second question: How complex or creative are your food tastes?

Some people have simple tastes in food and wine, while others are aware of and appreciate different layers of complexity. Maybe you're like several of my friends who can talk for a half hour about the delicate intricacies of a vintage wine. While they're swirling, smelling, and savoring a glass of wine, I can polish off a whole box of wine on my own.

Do you like to cook? Can you create your own dishes by experimenting with new combinations of ingredients? Gourmet chefs can spend a week planning a menu, picking recipes, shopping for ingredients, and so forth. Their creative investment in food is on an entirely different level than mine, which at best involves picking which take-out menu to order from or which frozen dinner to microwave.

Third question: Do you enjoy spicy food?

Being an aficionado of Taco Bell, not a day goes by that I'm not asked, "What kind of salsa would you like?" Some folks play it safe and order mild. Others like to live on the wild side and order extra hot. We each have our own spicy food comfort zone. Maybe you avoid spicy foods altogether, or maybe you are like several friends of mine who insist on ordering the hottest item on the menu.

Have you ever experimented with spicy food? How did it turn out? Maybe you stepped outside of your spicy food comfort zone and discovered you really liked flaming hot nachos or spicy Thai cuisine. Or maybe you're like me and got talked into eating a particularly hot chili pepper and still swear you can feel it tingling through your skull.

Are You Open to Expanding Your Sexual Diet?

Don't worry. You haven't accidentally picked up Rachel Ray's new cookbook. This is still a book about sex.

I asked you to think about your tastes in food and your openness to trying new things in this arena of your life because I think it helps to think about your sexual interests in the broader context of your life and all of your likes and dislikes. Some folks like to stick to routines and do this in every aspect of their life. Others like every day of their life to be a new adventure. Most of us fall somewhere in between.

People differ in the breadth of sexual activities they enjoy and their openness to sexual experimentation. In the next section, we'll take an inventory of your experiences and interests. Maybe you have a lot of sexual curiosity and will try anything once. Or maybe your tastes are more the meat-and-potatoes variety.

People also differ in their sexual creativity and complexity. Maybe you're completely satisfied with the same sexual menu week after week. Or maybe you're a sexual gourmet who loves to mix up various sexual ingredients to create new fantasies and scenarios to act out with your partner. Since I believe everyone's sexual diet could benefit from a little variety, I'll encourage you to sample new things and be a bit more creative. But I also understand that people with simple sexual tastes tend to view this as a lot of work. You are who you are, and there's nothing wrong with having simple sexual tastes.

My point is that we each have our own unique approach to sex, and it's best to keep labels, judgments, and expectations to a minimum. People who like really spicy food are not typical or average, but we don't label them as deviants. Similarly, people who like the spicier and kinkier side of sex also are not normal or mainstream, but there is also nothing intrinsically deviant in the kinky activities we'll explore in this chapter. If it's not your thing, that's fine. But if you venture outside your comfort zone, you may find some things that you really enjoy that are outside of your typical sexual diet.

The Range of Sexual Variety

Can We Count the Ways?

There are several ways we can gauge the breadth of your sexual interests and your openness to sexual experimentation. Over the years, I've come up with three questions that I believe do a pretty good job of sorting people into different levels of sexual adventurousness. We'll get to those in a moment, but let's start with doing things the old-fashioned way.

The most established method of assessing the range and scope of sexual interests is to use some form of sex inventory. As a rough indicator of your adventurousness, we can simply count up all the sexual activities you have tried or are open to trying.

The inventory I use was influenced by the granddaddy of all sex research, Alfred Kinsey. I went to graduate school at Indiana University, where he did his landmark research. One of the first things I did when I moved to Bloomington was go to the biology department and see where he used to lecture. For people who study human sexuality, this is holy ground.

When I was doing my dissertation research, I interviewed a woman who had been one of Dr. Kinsey's study participants. She had been nineteen years old at the time. She told me about how he had asked her questions for about an hour and written everything she said in a shorthand code on a single index card. Kinsey did about eleven thousand of these interviews on his own.[5]

I asked her what it was like to be asked such personal questions that must have been really shocking at the time (for example, Have you had an overt homosexual experience to the point of orgasm?). Her response to my question was, basically, Why should it have bothered me? He was a "doctor from the university," as she put it. "I knew he probably had a good reason to ask me about that sort of thing...and I knew he wasn't going to tell anyone what I said."

This Midwestern, no-nonsense attitude and trust for authority is pretty hard to find these days. There are few trusted institutions left in modern society. Most people are suspicious (and for good reasons) of the motives and confidentiality of questions about their sexual practices. So, unfortunately, even fifty years later, we still have a very incomplete picture of what constitutes the normal or typical range of human sexual activities.

In my own small way, I've tried to carry on in Kinsey's tradition by asking people straightforward questions about what they like to do sexually, how they do it, when and where, and so forth. I've included an abbreviated version of the inventory I use in Exercise 1.

Exercise 1: Inventory of Sexual Interests and Activities		
✓ = Yes ✗ = No ? = Unsure	Have You Done This?	Will You in the Future?
WHO You Have Sex With		
Have a no-strings-attached sexual fling		
Have anonymous sex		
Have sex with someone of same gender		
Have sex with someone of opposite gender		
Have sex with a transgender person		
Have a threesome		
Have a foursome		
Participate in an orgy		
Be watched while I masturbate		
Watch someone else masturbate		
Watch a couple having sex (via the Internet or webcam)		
Watch a couple having sex (while in the same room)		
Be watched while having sex with a partner		

WHAT You Do Sexually		
French kiss		
Make out		
Massage (or be massaged) as part of sex		
Striptease		
Kiss with champagne or other drink in your mouths		
Lick my partner's body		
Have my partner lick my body		
Be manually stimulated or masturbated by my partner		
Manually stimulate or masturbate my partner		
Receive oral sex		
Give oral sex		
69 (or simultaneous and mutual oral sex)		
Rim my partner (oral anal stimulation)		
Be rimmed by my partner		
Have vaginal intercourse		
Be anal intercourse top		
Be anal intercourse bottom		
Have intercourse in the missionary position		
Have intercourse "doggie style"		
Have intercourse while standing up		
Have intercourse in wild or unique positions		
Stick my finger inside my partner's butt		
Have my partner's finger inside my butt		
Fisted someone or been fisted		
Tug on my (or my partner's) balls or testicles		
Pinch my partner's nipples		
Have my nipples pinched		
Be spanked		
Spank my partner with my hand		
Be paddled		

Paddle my partner		
Shave (or be shaved by) my partner		
Take erotic pictures of or with my partner		
Be blindfolded		
Put a blindfold on my partner		
Be restrained with ropes, scarves, or handcuffs		
Restrain my partner with ropes, scarves, or handcuffs		
Use a "safe word" as part of sex		
Punish my partner in role-play		
WHERE You Have Sex		
Bedroom		
Bathroom		
Shower		
Bathtub		
Kitchen		
Living room		
Staircase		
Closet		
Home garage		
Home pool		
Home backyard		
In car parked at home driveway		
Office		
Workplace		
Public parking garage		
Other public place at risk of being caught		
Bar or nightclub		
Sex club or party		
Outdoors in a public park		

Outdoors on a camping trip or hike		
In a tent on a camping trip		
WHEN You Have Sex		
In the morning		
In the afternoon		
In the evening		
Middle of the night		
On a weekday or weeknight		
On a weekend		
Unplanned, surprise sex		
On vacation		
HOW You Have Sex		
Have slow and sensual sex		
Have gentle and tender sex		
Have fast and intense sex		
Have rough sex		
Change sexual positions multiple times		
Have sex with your clothes on		
Have sex while wearing costumes		
Be submissive to a partner		
Dominate my partner		
Take turns being dominant or submissive		
WHY You Have Sex		
To express love		
To express affection		
To have fun or be playful		
To be spiritually close to my partner		
To release stress		
To escape from the "real" world and pressures		

As fun as it would be to catalog every possible sexual activity, I chose to include only the most popular activities, plus a few exotic or spicy options. There are certainly lots of other resources you can explore if you want to do a really thorough inventory, starting with the *Kama Sutra.* Even Wikipedia has evolved into a pretty thorough compendium of sexual activities. So if you noticed I didn't include "the Italian Banker" or a "rusty trombone" in my inventory, you can always look it up there.

So take a moment to complete Exercise 1. I organized the options under variations in who, what, where, when, how, and why you have sex. For each activity, there are two questions: Have you done this activity? Are you interested in doing this in the future? Use a ✓ for yes, an ✗ for no, or a ? for unsure. We'll look at the pattern of these marks across the two columns to get a sense of your overall sexual adventurousness.

What's on Your Wish List?

Everyone has a list of sexual favorites. You probably also have a wish list of things you would like to try someday or are at least curious about. Perhaps you have a "no way" list of things that are too weird, too complicated, too painful, or too gross for you to ever even consider trying.

We can translate the inventory in Exercise 1 into something similar to these lists by looking at the pattern of your ratings in the "have done it" versus "will do it" columns. Basically, every item in the sexual universe can potentially be sorted into

✓✓ Done it and would like to do it again.

✓✗ Done it and will not do it again.

✗✓ Haven't yet but definitely want to.

✗? Haven't yet but am curious.

✗✗ Haven't yet nor do I ever want to do.

Which Pattern Describes You Best?

Looking over your ratings in the inventory, which combination of ratings was most common? Depending on which of these five pairings was most prominent in your inventory, this is what it tells you about your sexual interests:

- ✓✓ *Sexual Adventurers:* If you look down the two columns in Exercise 1 and see all ✓✓, it means you have tried almost everything and plan to do it all again. Obviously, you are very sexually adventurous. You should probably consider writing your own book.

- ✓✗ *Sexually Focused:* If the left column is filled with ✓s paired with ✗s in the right column, then you've obviously been around the block a few times. But, for whatever reason, you don't plan on visiting those same activities again. Maybe they were fun at one time in your life, but now that you've sown your wild oats, you're ready to settle down. Or perhaps you spent a lot of time experimenting before you found a set of activities that you enjoyed.

- ✗✓ *Sexual Explorers:* If you don't have a lot of sexual experience, or at least lack a variety of experiences, then you have a lot of ✗s in the left column. If you filled most of the right column with ✓s, then you are what I call a sexual explorer. You are looking to expand your sexual repertoire and expect to enjoy a wide variety of sexual play in the future. Even if you're not sure you'd like something, you're committed to giving everything a try at least once.

✗? *Sexually Curious:* If you have a lot of ✗s in the left column and mostly question marks in right column, then you are very curious about sex but not sure whether you'll ever act on your curiosity.

✗✗ *Sexually Conservative:* If you filled both columns of Exercise 1 with ✗s, then you have a relatively narrow set of sexual experiences and are satisfied with your favorite set of activities.

We'll come back to these descriptions at the end of the chapter, when we look at the big picture of your sexual adventurousness. The quantity of your sexual interests is definitely part of the story, but it's not the whole story. We also need to factor in your overall sexual creativity and your openness to the darker and kinkier aspects of sex.

But before we get to these, let's take a quick look at how most men and women have responded to this inventory and what seems to constitute typical and atypical sexual interests. Let's look at differences in where, when, and how people like to have sex.

Where Do You Like to Have Sex?

Obviously, the most common locale for sex is the bedroom. The next most popular home setting is in the bathroom (in the shower or tub). Occasionally a couple will brag about having sex in front of their fireplace, but it's actually pretty rare for a couple to have sex outside of their bedroom. Among the places people say they would most like to have sex is on an airplane (a.k.a., the Mile High Club), outdoors, and somewhere in public but hidden out of view.

When Do You Like to Have Sex?

In case you haven't noticed, the most common time for sex is during the evening. Morning sex is the next most popular, followed by sex during the day on Saturday or Sunday. Sex outside of these time windows is so rare that if you have sex on a weekday afternoon, you're practically a sexual weirdo.

Most couples say they have sex at a regular or planned time each week, every other week, or at another routine interval. One of the most commonly picked activities that both men and women say they would like to do more often is have surprise sex. It's unplanned, unscripted, and a little naughty. Unfortunately, the longer a couple has been together, the less likely that they report having spontaneous or impulsive sex.

How Do You Like to Have Sex?

Most individuals and couples have a preferred way they like for sex to unfold. Most couples say they follow a standard sequence, which is similar to the common baseball analogy, starting with first base (kissing), followed by second base (fondling), etc.[6] They also tend to be pretty consistent about how much time is given to each activity.

On average, new couples spend about forty minutes having sex; long-term couples spend about fifteen to twenty minutes. If you have a low need for sexual variety, you probably dedicate about the same amount of time for each sexual encounter. However, couples who like to mix things up sexually enjoy both long and short sessions. Sometimes they take the time to set the mood, light candles, take a bubble bath, and so forth. Other times they enjoy a fast, frenzied quickie.

Two other variations in how sex unfolds are worth mentioning. First, people differ in how much they prefer to *give* versus *receive* sexually. Most men and women say they enjoy both. However, when forced to choose one or the other, most women say they prefer to give, and most men say they prefer to receive. Indeed, more women than men say they feel uncomfortable being the focus of their partner's attention.

Second, people differ in how much they like to take the lead sexually versus follow their partner's lead. Which do you prefer? Do you like to be the one who chooses or initiates which activities are tried, for how long, in which order, and at what pace?

Preferences vary widely in this arena, although most men and women expect someone to take charge sexually. About one in three men (29 percent) and women (34 percent) prefer a traditional gender dynamic where the *man* takes the sexual initiative and plays an assertive role sexually. About one in four men (27 percent) and one in five women (21 percent) say they prefer a dynamic where the *woman* takes the lead and the man lets her shape how sex unfolds. The remaining women (26 percent) and men (15 percent) say they prefer a relationship where neither partner takes the lead or both take the lead equally.

Although it seems like this equal sharing of control during sex would be the ideal arrangement, having no one in charge appears to come with some risks. More egalitarian couples are more likely to stick to a sexual routine and have relatively little variety in their sex lives. Apparently, in order to try new things and mix up the flow of sex, it helps to have one partner who takes the wheel and guides the experience.

To sum up, the more you like to mix up the *sequence* of what you do first, second, and so forth, and the more you vary who *gives* and who *receives,* and who *takes the lead* and who *follows,* the more variety you have in your sex life.

Now that we've cataloged your sexual interests, let's shift gears a bit and look at two other approaches to gauging your sexual adventurousness. Let's look at how much creativity you bring to sex in general. Then we'll take a closer look at the kinkier side of sex.

Sexual Creativity

Is Sex a Playful Experience?

Making love is the most common and socially acceptable form of sex. But sex can also be a way to connect with someone on a playful and physical level. To say that sex can *only* be satisfying when it's in the context of love and emotional intimacy excludes whole categories of sexual experiences within relationships (and outside of relationships) that center around fun, play, and creativity. For single men and women, these experiences are often exciting and satisfying precisely because they are free from emotional involvement and expectations. For couples, playful sex can be a way to set aside their roles as spouses, roommates, or parents and try on new roles and personalities.

Do You Role-Play?

For some, sex is the ultimate creative experience. In Part 3, we'll look in depth at your inner sex life and your sexual fantasies. People with creative sex lives find ways to bring these fantasies to life through sexual role-play. As we'll see in Chapters 9 and 12, sexual role-play is typically built around two core themes. The first is power. One person often plays a dominant, powerful figure, while the other plays a more passive and submissive role. The second theme is the overall emotional tone, which can either be positive (light, innocent, and fun) or negative (dark, edgy, and nasty).

A wide variety of creative sexual experiences can be generated from these two themes. In Part 4, we'll look at the most popular role-play scenarios creative couples enjoy. They include highly structured scenarios (like seducing the plumber or playing a call girl) and more adventurous sexual play (like being blindfolded). But role-play can also be more informal and improvisational.

Formal role-play scenarios (like dressing up as a French maid) are like theatrical plays or orchestrated concerts, while informal role-play is more like jazz music. I have no musical talent myself, but I am told that musicians feel a real rush while creating music together and playing off one another's ideas and impulses. Sex with a creative partner can be like this as well.

Being very verbal during sex or talking dirty can generate informal roles. Any time a lover says, "I wish we were…" or "Remember the time when we…," he or she is pulling sex out of normal reality and into a more playful experience.

Do You Have Good Improvisational Skills?

People who are sexually creative are like improvisational actors. They instinctively know how to encourage the flow of sex and let it go to new and interesting places.

I took an improvisational acting class in college. The only thing I remember from it is the so-called *yes-and* rule. When you're improvising a scene with a partner, you always answer any question your partner throws at you with "yes" and then build on it. You usually have no idea where your partner is going, but you say yes to keep the momentum going and then add something of your own to the flow. If you say no, it throws up a roadblock, and things quickly fall apart.

If you're a creative lover, you probably do the same thing as part of sex and always accept and add to your lover's creative instincts. If your lover wants to talk dirty, for example, you can easily pick up on this and run with it.

In sum, if you are turned on by structured role-play scenarios or even informal sexual role-play, then your sexual tastes are more complex and creative than most men and women. Only about one in three men and women regularly incorporate role-play into sex. However, over half of all men and women say they are curious about role-play and would like to be more playful during sex. So Parts 3 and 4 of the book offer a road map for transforming your sex life from simple and predictable to creative and surprising.

Kinky Sex

Are You Kinky?

I've come to believe that kinky is in the eye of the beholder. Years ago, when my colleague Dr. Glenn Hutchinson did our first sex surveys on the Internet, we were shocked to learn how many men and women described themselves as kinky. As we dug deeper and deeper into what people really meant by kinky, we learned that in most cases saying you were kinky was a way of saying that (1) you liked sex and (2) you were open to trying out new sexual positions and activities.

A person with kinky tastes was anyone who was a little more sexually adventurous than you. If you always had sex in the missionary position, for example, sex standing up was seen as kinky.

Over time, I've narrowed down a set of fifteen sexual activities that most people see as kinky that still remain outside of the mainstream of sexual experience. I've listed these activities in Exercise 2. The kinkiest items on the list tend to involve sex that is mixed with pain, fear, or danger.

Take a moment to rate how interested you are in each of these activities from 1 (not at all interested) to 9 (very interested). If you add up your ratings, you can compare your total with other people who have taken the inventory. As a rule, if you are very interested in at least nine or ten of the activities, then you can feel confident in describing yourself as kinky.

Why Are Some People Kinkier than Others?

I believe three factors push some individuals to want and seek out very novel and intense sexual experiences. The first is pleasure. Almost all of the activities in Exercises 1 and 2 are physically pleasurable in some way. So it makes sense that the more of them you try, the more fun you have. As Mae West once said, "Too much of a good thing... is wonderful."

As I mentioned in the previous chapter, the very act of seeking out and exploring new experiences and sensations can itself be pleasurable. The brain's reward system releases stimulating chemicals, which make seeing, touching, and interacting with new things enjoyable. I imagine some individuals receive more pleasure from sexual exploration than others.

The second factor that pushes some men and women toward kinky and adventurous sex is *habituation.* In general, our minds tend to habituate to new experiences. The more often you encounter the same situation, the more your reactions turn into habits. Each time you visit the same place or meet the same person again, for example, your mind takes in less information. Your mind isn't lazy; it's simply efficient. It doesn't waste energy sensing or feeling things when it already knows what to expect.

Habituation can be a big obstacle for couples trying to maintain a satisfying long-term sex life. There's a big difference between all the surprises and sensations you experience the first time you have sex with someone and the one hundredth time. No matter what you do, sex with your monogamous partner will tend to get more predictive over time.

Not everyone is affected by habituation in the same way. Some people seem to be more prone to boredom and habituation than others. Some folks can enjoy the same sexual menu again and again, while others become habituated very quickly. For them, familiarity may not breed contempt, but it certainly breeds disinterest.[7]

The third factor that pushes some individuals to seek out kinky sex is a desire to use sex as a means of distraction and *escape.* It turns out that habituation not only interferes with our ability to enjoy sex, it also reduces the intensity of the experience. It can make it harder and harder for sex to work as a way to let off steam.

Exercise 2: Kinky Sex Inventory

How interested are you in these activities? Place your 1 to 9 ratings in the circles. Then, sum your ratings.

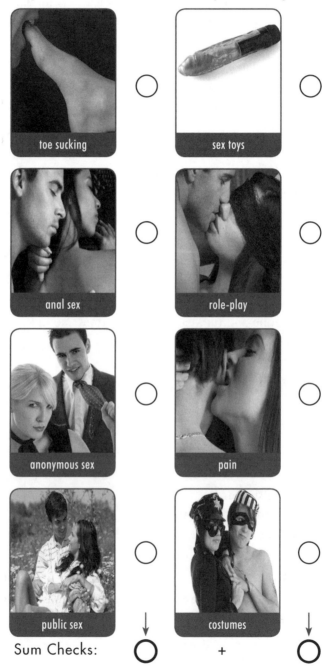

toe sucking

sex toys

anal sex

role-play

anonymous sex

pain

public sex

costumes

Sum Checks: +

Not at All
Interested

① ② ③ ④ ⑤ ⑥ ⑦ ⑧ ⑨

Very
Interested

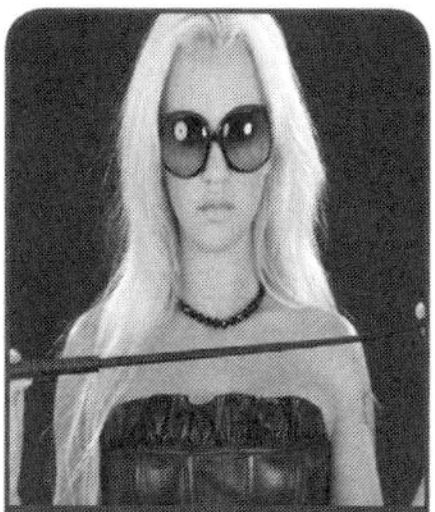

punishment

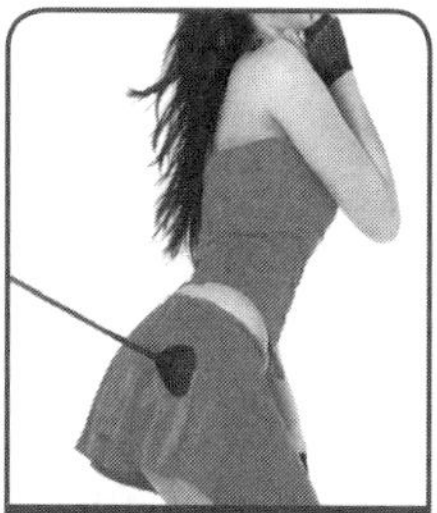

○

spanking

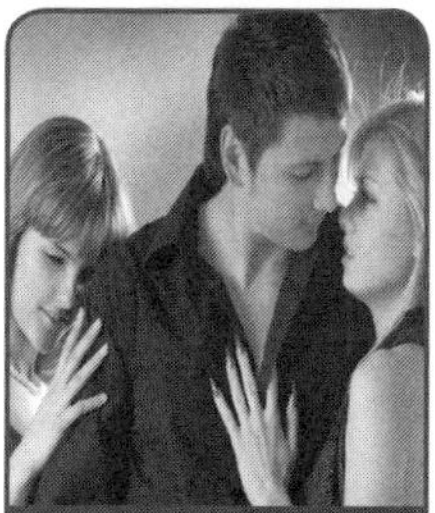

○

threesome

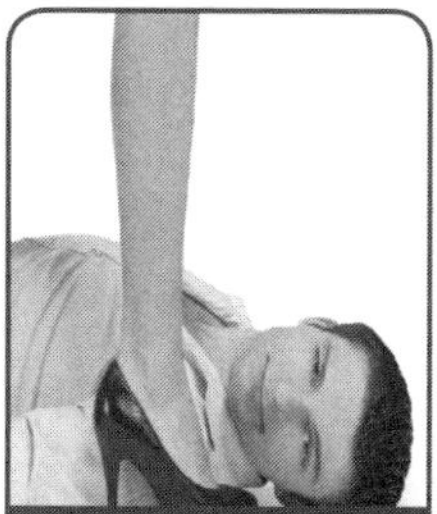

○

fetish play

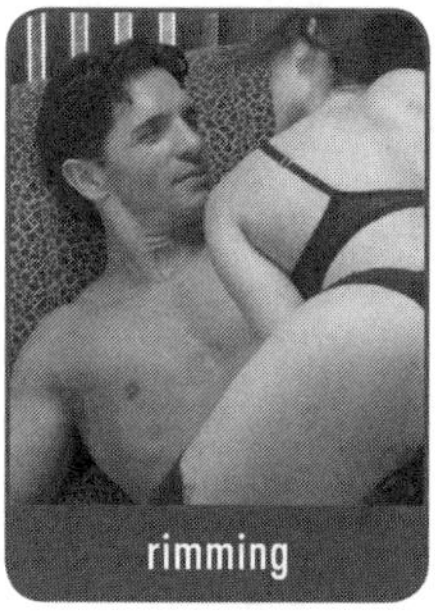

○

KEY:

< 25 = Very
Low

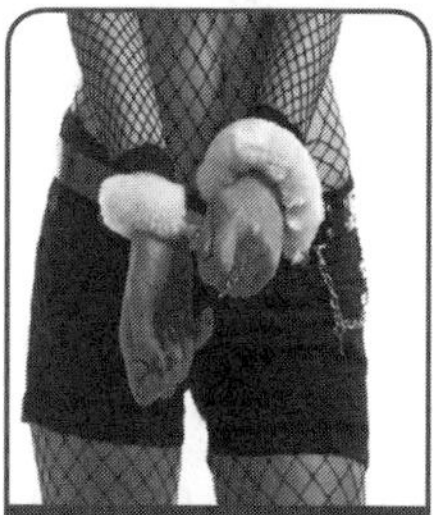

25–45 = Low

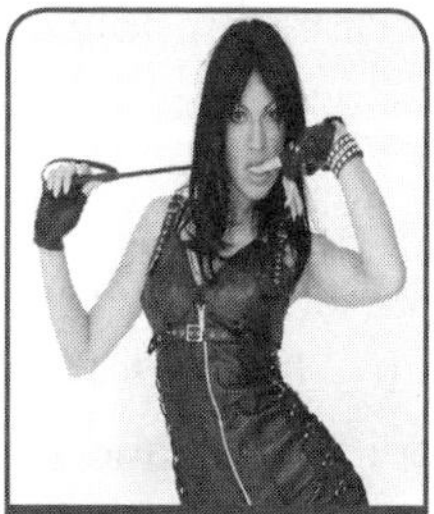

45–75 =
Average

75–95 = High

95+ = Very
High

rimming

○

bondage

○

leather

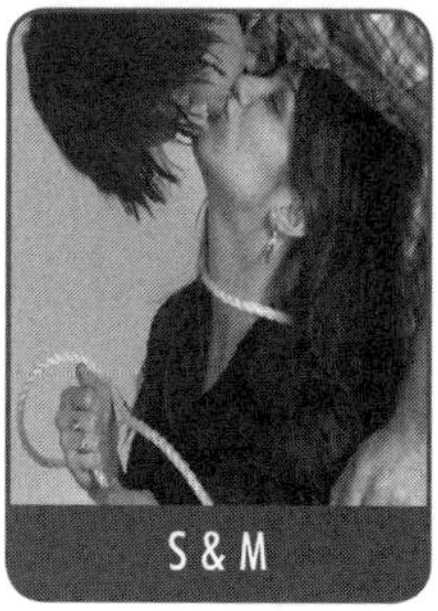

+

↓
○

S & M

+

↓
○ = ☐

Oftentimes, the more intense your stressors and worries, the more intense the counteremotional experience will need to be in order to distract you. This is probably why you occasionally hear about high-power CEOs who like to be whipped or punished by a dominatrix. They have to seek out more and more intense sensations in order to drown out their work pressures and other worries.

To sum up, I think it's important to understand not only what you like sexually but why you like it, especially when it comes to kinky sex. If you are seeking new and more intense sexual experiences because you are easily bored, then you and your partner are going to have to make an ongoing commitment to mix things up sexually. The challenge is to stay one step ahead of your tendency to habituate and mix things up *before* you get bored.

Categories of Adventurousness

Which Category Describes Your Tastes?

You are the only one who knows enough about your sexual interests to put a name or label on your tastes. I'm a little cautious about throwing labels like kinky or adventurous around, because they tend to lump together and oversimplify people's sexual experiences. But for whatever reason, people tend to be curious about these labels and want to know how their tastes compare to other men and women. I see nothing wrong with using labels like Vanilla or Kinky, especially if they can help you understand your own sexuality or communicate with your partner about what you want from your sex life.

I've developed a system for sorting people into four categories from Vanilla to Kinky by using the series of options mapped out in Exercise 3. The labels at the bottom of this chart are not definitive and absolute. But I hope you can use them as a tool to explore your interests and see whether the category you end up in fits. If you have a partner, you can go through the exercise with his or her interests in mind as well.

The exercise centers on the three dimensions of sexual variety we've reviewed in this chapter:

- Variety in sexual activities (what you like to do, when, where, and how)
- Sexual creativity and the extent to which you like to use fantasy and role-play as part of sex
- Your interests in kinky sex

It starts by presenting three options (sex with handcuffs, sex blindfolded, and sex in a shower) and asks which sexual activity you've tried and enjoyed. Based on my research, if you've had sex with handcuffs and enjoyed it, then you can skip the rest of the exercise, because you almost certainly have kinky tastes. If you haven't tried any of these activities and haven't even had sex in a shower, then you probably have Vanilla tastes. The rest of you have two more sets of options to explore, and your placement depends on how much sexual variety you enjoy and whether you have tried (and enjoyed) rough sex, role-play sex, or sex that involves pain.

How Common Are Vanilla versus Kinky Tastes?

Let's take a quick look at each of the four categories. For efficiency's sake, I've summarized each category by using feminine pronouns, but the categories apply to both men and women. I also describe how many men and women fall into each of the categories, which is also presented in Figure 1.

A person with Vanilla sexual tastes enjoys the sexual basics: kissing, some oral foreplay, and intercourse. She has a sexual routine

Exercise 3: How Sexually Adventurous Are You?

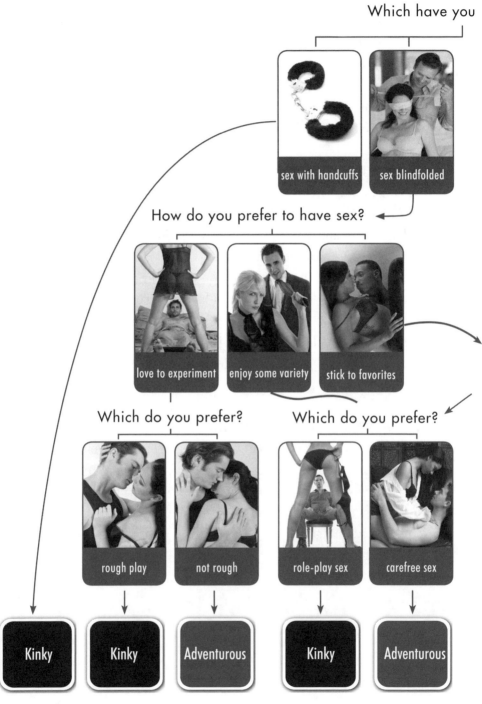

tried and enjoyed?

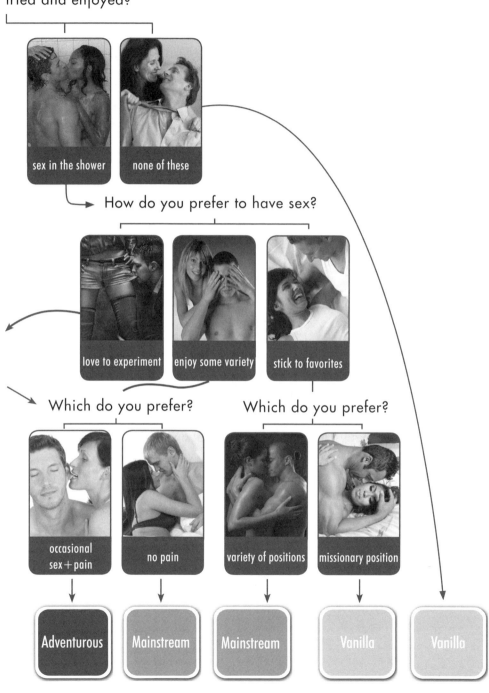

and is not interested in changing when and where she has sex. She has a favorite position for intercourse (usually missionary) and is not interested in other positions. She tends to prefer traditional power dynamics, with the same partner taking the lead each time, and one partner being somewhat more dominant than the other. She is not interested in any form of sex that involves pain, fear, or anything weird or complicated.

In the inventory at the start of the chapter (Exercise 1), people with Vanilla tastes were probably labeled sexually conservative because they had lots of *X*'s on all the activities they had not tried and had no interest in trying. Only about one in ten men fall in the Vanilla category. Twice as many women have Vanilla tastes, but that's still only one in five.

To say a person has mainstream tastes implies three things. First, her current sexual practices center on the sexual basics and usually follow a preferred routine of when, where, and how sex unfolds.

Second, although she may be curious about adventurous activities (such as sex toys, bondage, and anal sex), she has no or limited experience trying them out. So some of the sexually curious individuals from Exercise 1 may end up in the mainstream category and will stay there unless they actually branch out and experiment more with sex.

Third, the emotional tone of her sexual experiences is usually positive, carefree, and fun. She is not interested in exploring darker sexual fantasies or role-play. About half of all men and women have mainstream tastes.

A person with Adventurous sexual tastes enjoys experimenting with new and different sexual positions and activities. She becomes bored with the same sexual routine. In fact, if she had her way, she would never have sex in the exact same way twice. She has an active fantasy life, enjoys sexual role-play, and likes to mix up power dynamics with her partner. Although she's open to trying activities that may involve a little pain (like pinching nipples or spanking), she does so primarily to surprise her partner and keep sex exciting. Pain or a dark emotional tone can add to sexual variety, but is not a requirement.

About one in five women and one in four men fall into the Adventurous group.

Age differences in sexual interests are relatively small. The likelihood of having Adventurous tastes climbs a little bit starting in the late twenties and peaks at about age fifty in my studies.

To say a person has Kinky tastes usually implies three things. First, she enjoys a relatively narrow set of sexual activities that are outside of Mainstream sexual tastes. In fact, most other people view their interests (such as fetishes, punishment, and masochism) as weird or bizarre.

Having kinky sexual tastes does not necessarily mean the individual has a wide variety of sexual interests. Many of the sexually focused individuals from Exercise 1 end up in the Kinky category. If, for example, the only way you can have an orgasm is with a gag in your mouth and a six-inch stiletto on your back, then your sexual interests are about as narrow as they get.

Second, fantasy and role-play are central to most sexual encounters. Sex without creative scenarios or specific power dynamics is viewed as boring and predictable. Third, the emotional tone of the sexual experience is usually dark and incorporates pain, fear, or danger as a way to intensify the experience.

Only about one in seven men and women have Kinky tastes. Slightly more men than women fall into the Adventurous and Kinky categories, but it's not a huge difference.

Do You Want a Partner Who Is More Adventurous?

The majority of men and women say they want a partner who has similar sexual interests and a similar need for sexual variety. However, about one in four people say they would prefer a partner who is *more* adventurous than they are. Interestingly, this trend exists among both women and men.[8]

In a way, wanting a partner who is more sexually adventurous is itself a sign of adventurousness. Therefore, in an obvious attempt to blow my mind, a number of the men and women in my studies have described themselves as being sexually Mainstream but then turned around and said they wanted a partner who is sexually adventurous. Oftentimes, these men and women would fit in the sexually curious category from Exercise 1. They want to experiment sexually, but thus far they haven't had a partner who was open to trying new things.

Do Sexually Adventurous People Have Higher Sex Drives?

It turns out that sex drive and sexual adventurousness are closely connected. In Figure 1, I listed for each of the Adventurous categories the proportion of men and women with high or very high sex drives.

The vast majority of men and women with Vanilla or Mainstream tastes have low or moderate sex drives. Among people with Vanilla tastes, for example, only about one in ten like to have sex every day. I guess if you have relatively simple sexual tastes, you don't tend to like to eat from that menu every single day.

In contrast, about half of the men and women with Adventurous

Figure 1: Levels of Sexual Adventurousness

	% of Women	% of Men	% High Sex Drive
Vanilla	21%	11%	13%
Mainstream	46%	49%	18%
Adventurous	20%	24%	42%
Kinky	13%	16%	54%

 and = Approximately 10%

or Kinky tastes have high or very high sex drives. It's hard to disentangle which comes first. But it makes sense that someone who likes to have a lot of sex would also need to mix things up sexually in order to avoid becoming habituated to the same experience over and over again.

As we'll see in Part 2, this has implications for deciding who you should have sex with and especially for finding a compatible long-term partner. Your chances of finding what you want depend on which combination of sex drive and sexual adventurousness you are looking for. It's easier to find a partner with a low sex drive and Vanilla tastes than it is to find a partner with a high sex drive and Vanilla tastes, for example. So let's turn to what you can do to either find the basics of sexual compatibility in a new partner or create a compatible balance in your existing relationship.

PART 2

How Can You Find (or Create) Sexual Compatibility?

Chapter 3

Clues That Reveal
Sexual Compatibility

Judging Compatibility

What's Next for Single Folks?

In Part 1, we started to paint a picture of the type of sex life you want to have and the type of lover who would best match your sex drive and interests. In this chapter, we'll look at steps you can take to find a partner who shares these basics of sexual compatibility. If you're already in a relationship, you may want to skip to the next chapter, where we look at ways to reignite your sexual spark with your current partner.

Having designed matchmaking systems for over a decade, I've given a lot of thought to the challenges single men and women face as they search for compatible partners. Along the way, I've learned a number of clues you can watch for that can help you anticipate whether or not someone might be a good fit. If nothing else, these clues can prompt you to ask questions and explore whether or not the two of you share similar sexual goals *before* you have sex or at least before you develop a deep emotional connection.

But first I want to offer a few words of caution to single folks. I want to encourage you to be skeptical when you see or hear advertisements from websites and matchmakers that promise to find your "perfect match." Although it would be comforting to believe that technology and science could take the guesswork out of dating, the truth is that there are inherent limits to how well we can predict compatibility both in and out of the bedroom.

Can You Predict Compatibility Before You Meet?

When I worked with dating websites like Match.com and Yahoo!, I was an outspoken critic of websites like eHarmony.com and Chemistry.com that promised to deliver soul mates and spouses. The Internet can be an efficient and effective way to meet new people and expand the scope of your dating options. But sites that promise (or imply) they can find you a husband or wife go too far in my opinion. In the research I have done, I've found that these sorts of sites consistently overpromise and underdeliver.

Sites like eHarmony say they know the secret formula for predicting compatibility. They refer to research that shows that married couples with similar interests and values tend to be more satisfied. So they measure interests and values, and then they match people who are similar. However, the importance of a couple's similarities or differences depends enormously on *how* they manage their relationship.[9] There are plenty of couples with lots in common who are miserable, and there are many pairs of opposites who are blissfully happy.

When two people create a life together, the synergy of their relationship is more than the sum of their parts. The best predictors of marital satisfaction and the risk of divorce have to do with the way a couple communicates and manages conflict. However, you can only measure these sorts of dynamics *after* a couple is together.[10] There is no research to suggest we can measure something about two individuals *before* they meet that will tell us how well they would work out as a couple.

You should also be wary of any website that offers to predict marital compatibility based on a personality test. I like personality tests. I include an abbreviated personality test as an exercise in this chapter. I've also had success in using personality tests online to help pair individuals who would be a good match for *dating.* But my colleagues and I have never expected a personality test could predict who should or should not get married.[11]

Even if you had billions of dollars and all the resources in the world at your fingertips, you could never come up with a system that could identify who you should marry. Let's say you came up with a sophisticated laboratory test that could identify pairs of individuals who should *not* get married (because they would likely get divorced). Let's assume your ability to predict divorce was extremely accurate, more accurate than screening tests like mammograms or Pap smears. Even then, you would inevitably make more false predictions (predicting a divorce that would never happen) than true predictions (accurately foreseeing a divorce).[12]

So should we just give up on evaluating compatibility? No. We all make predictions about whom to go out with, whom to have sex with, and which relationships are worth pursuing. So we might as well do our best to make informed decisions that take into account as much relevant information as we can gather. But the person in charge of these decisions needs to be *you,* not some bogus website that pretends to know your needs and desires better than you do.

What Clues Can You Watch For?

In this chapter we'll look at one potential set of clues to watch for when judging compatibility both inside and outside of the bedroom. We'll start by reviewing the personality types you find attractive.

Then we'll look at the link between personality traits and sexual interests. We'll see how traits such as shyness, intelligence, dependability, and niceness may offer clues to a potential date's sex drive and sexual adventurousness. You can't always judge a book by its cover, but knowing the connection between sexual interests and personality can help you anticipate where to invest your dating energies and some of the trade-offs you may face in finding Mr. or Ms. Right (or Mr. or Ms. Right Now).

Personality Attraction

Are Sex Symbols Always Beautiful?

A big part of what makes someone sexy is his or her personality. Many of the great lovers and sex symbols from history and literature were exceptional primarily because of who they were and how they acted, rather than how they looked.

Cleopatra is portrayed as one of history's great beauties. Indeed, she beguiled and seduced both Julius Caesar and Marc Antony. However, judging from descriptions of her in letters as well as a coin from that period that shows a profile of her face, her facial features were not especially beautiful. What made her so compelling were her many interests and talents. She was fluent in at least seven languages and was an exceptional conversationalist. Caesar commented that she was the only woman he ever met whom he could talk to as an equal.

If you've ever watched the 1939 film *Gone with the Wind*, it's hard to separate the character of Scarlett O'Hara from the stunningly beautiful actress Vivien Leigh. So it may surprise you to learn that Margaret Mitchell's 1932 *book* opens with: "Scarlett O'Hara was not beautiful, but men seldom realized it when caught by her charm." The book goes on to describe how both men and women were entranced by Scarlett's provocative personality and passion for life.

So, what is it that can make even an ordinary looking man or woman incredibly sexy? Why is it that you can be very physically attracted to someone but then lose all interest in him or her after even a brief conversation?

The answer lies in the mysteries of personality attraction. Let's look at the specific combination of personality traits you tend to find most compelling and attractive.

Why Talk about Personality Types?

For years, my collaborator Glenn Hutchinson and I resisted using personality-type lingo. It's hard to pigeonhole people into a set of narrow types, since how people describe themselves changes a fair amount from day to day and from situation to situation. If you ask someone to describe how he acts, thinks, and feels at work and then ask the same questions focused on his social life, you'll probably get a different set of answers.

Still, personality lingo has come to play a pretty big role in our culture and how we view ourselves. It also plays a big role in how we describe other people. For better or for worse, personality labels have taken on even more meaning in the Internet age as a shorthand way of labeling ourselves and our interests.

So Glenn and I, working with our great team of research assistants and academic advisors, spent several years developing a typology of personality traits. We looked at over seven hundred possible combinations of traits that people tended to find attractive. Fortunately, some combinations were more common than others. Men who are attracted to outgoing and sociable women, for example, tend to also be interested in women who are open-minded and like to try new things. Men who are drawn to more shy and introverted women, in contrast, usually want a more traditional and conservative partner.

For our matchmaking system on Yahoo!, we created twelve primary types, each with three subtypes (for a total of thirty-six types). Over 90 percent of the people who used the system on Yahoo! said their type description fit their personality.

Now, for the purposes of this book, I'm going to trim down the types even further to eight *public personas.* I'm sure Glenn will belt me with eggs for oversimplifying things, and he will be right to do so. But I decided to use a set of types that I could communicate in a simple chart. The eight types still cover about 80 percent of the most common types people identify with and 85 percent of the types men and women tend to find attractive.

So I hope you find the exercises in the next section helpful. I refer to these types throughout the book as a shorthand way to talk about our public personalities and how these often differ from our sexual personalities. However, keep in mind that they are just tools. Use the labels if they're helpful, but throw them out if they get in the way of understanding the complexities of who you are and who you find attractive.

Which Personality Type Do You Find Most Appealing?

Take a look at either Exercise 1 or 2 to explore the public persona you find most attractive. Then complete the exercise with photos of your own gender to see which persona best describes your own personality.

There are three branches, and each choice presents two contrasting traits or personal qualities. You can either follow the branches in the chart or look at the descriptive words that summarize each type at the bottom of the chart. I suggest you do both. Remember these are rough tools. If none of the personas describe you or describe the type you find attractive, try looking at the results for several personas. You may be a unique case who is best described by a combination of personas or is looking for a unique combination.

Like most people, you probably hate being forced to choose between two options, especially if you like both choices or dislike both of them. Nevertheless, trust your initial gut reaction and see where it leads you. If it's a toss-up between the options, go down both pathways and see which outcome is the best fit.

What Are the Most Common Personality Types?

Based on research using charts like these as well as studies using more sophisticated sorting tools, I have estimated the percentage of men and women who fall into the eight public personas. These are mapped out in Figure 1 for women and Figure 2 for men.

The five most common types among both men and women are *traditional, smart, faithful, grounded,* and *nice.* Women are more likely to fit in the *traditional* and *grounded* types, while men are more likely to fit in the *smart* and *faithful* types. The three *least* common types are *rebel, adventurer,* and *shy.*

What Are the Most Popular Personality Types?

Each of the public personas is appealing in its own way.[13] Each has its own target audience or fan base.

In Figures 1 and 2, I've listed for each public persona (1) the percentage of men and women who find the type very or extremely attractive and (2) the percentage who find the type very or extremely *un*attractive.

The closest we come to a universally attractive personality type is the Nice persona. About two out of three men and women find this persona very or extremely attractive. Very few adults find this type to be unappealing. So, at least when it comes to public personas, nice guys (and gals) finish first.

There is no universally unattractive public persona. This is partly by design, since I intentionally selected personas that were both common and popular. Nevertheless, the Shy persona is the least popular of the options included here. Only 6 percent of women find

Exercise 1: FEMALE Public Persona

Which trait describes you

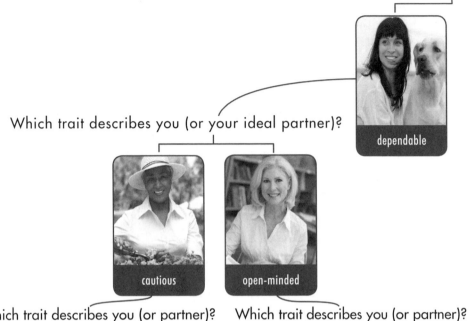

dependable

Which trait describes you (or your ideal partner)?

cautious

open-minded

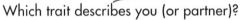

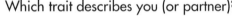

Which trait describes you (or partner)?

Which trait describes you (or partner)?

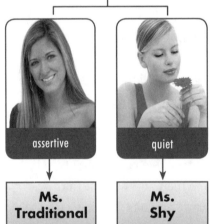

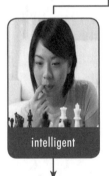

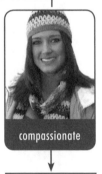

assertive

quiet

intelligent

compassionate

Ms. **Traditional**	Ms. **Shy**	Ms. **Smart**	Ms. **Faithful**
Confident, Conservative, Reliable, Decent, Competitive, Hardworking, Decisive	Gentle, Reliable, Introverted, Neat, Private, Mild-Mannered, Calm, Reserved	Creative, Original, Tolerant, Goal Oriented, Conversational, Sophisticated, Honest, Talented	Friendly, Mature, Accepting, Polite, Idealistic, Sociable, Loyal, Gracious, Caring, Patient

(or your ideal partner)?

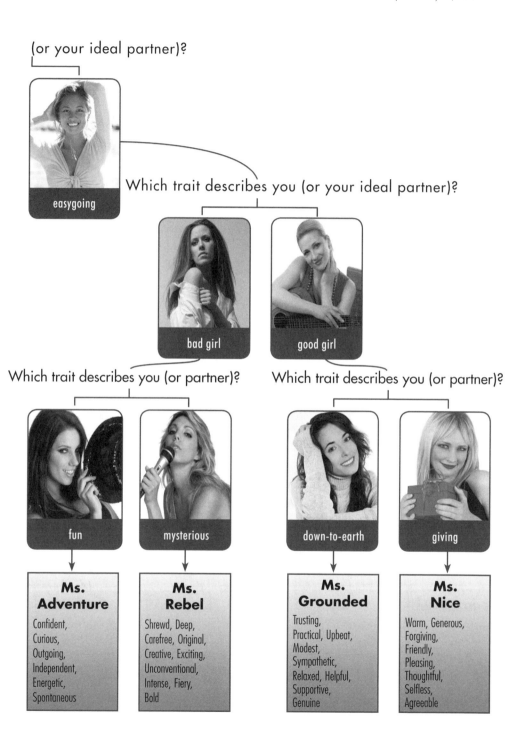

easygoing

Which trait describes you (or your ideal partner)?

bad girl

good girl

Which trait describes you (or partner)?

Which trait describes you (or partner)?

fun

mysterious

down-to-earth

giving

Ms. Adventure

Confident,
Curious,
Outgoing,
Independent,
Energetic,
Spontaneous

Ms. Rebel

Shrewd, Deep,
Carefree, Original,
Creative, Exciting,
Unconventional,
Intense, Fiery,
Bold

Ms. Grounded

Trusting,
Practical, Upbeat,
Modest,
Sympathetic,
Relaxed, Helpful,
Supportive,
Genuine

Ms. Nice

Warm, Generous,
Forgiving,
Friendly,
Pleasing,
Thoughtful,
Selfless,
Agreeable

Exercise 2: MALE Public Persona

Which trait describes you

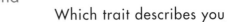

dependable

Which trait describes you (or your ideal partner)?

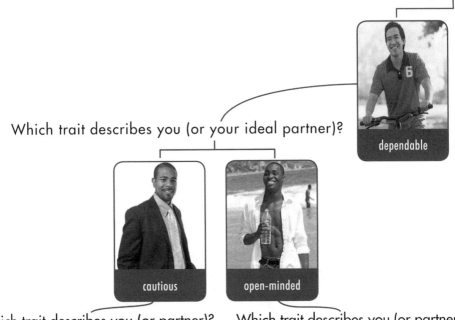

cautious   open-minded

Which trait describes you (or partner)?   Which trait describes you (or partner)?

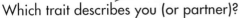

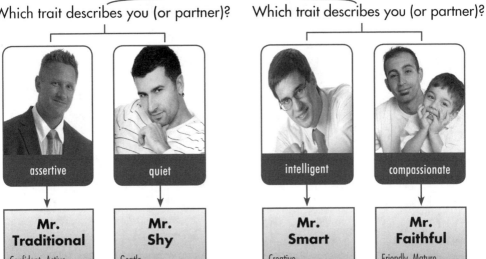

assertive   quiet   intelligent   compassionate

Mr. Traditional	Mr. Shy	Mr. Smart	Mr. Faithful
Confident, Active, Conservative, Reliable, Decent, Competitive, Hardworking, Decisive	Gentle, Reliable, Introverted, Neat, Private, Mild-Mannered, Calm, Reserved	Creative, Original, Goal Oriented, Conversational, Tolerant, Clever, Logical, Honest	Friendly, Mature, Accepting, Polite, Idealistic, Sociable, Caring, Chivalrous, Loyal, Patient

(or your ideal partner)?

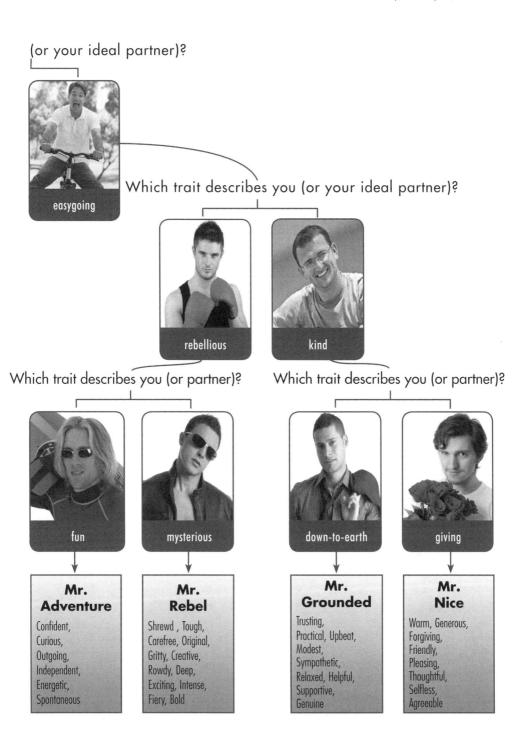

easygoing

Which trait describes you (or your ideal partner)?

rebellious

kind

Which trait describes you (or partner)?

Which trait describes you (or partner)?

fun

mysterious

down-to-earth

giving

Mr. Adventure

Confident,
Curious,
Outgoing,
Independent,
Energetic,
Spontaneous

Mr. Rebel

Shrewd , Tough,
Carefree, Original,
Gritty, Creative,
Rowdy, Deep,
Exciting, Intense,
Fiery, Bold

Mr. Grounded

Trusting,
Practical, Upbeat,
Modest,
Sympathetic,
Relaxed, Helpful,
Supportive,
Genuine

Mr. Nice

Warm, Generous,
Forgiving,
Friendly,
Pleasing,
Thoughtful,
Selfless,
Agreeable

Figure 1: Proportion of Women with Each Public Persona and Their Popularity

	% of Women	Men Who Find Her Attractive	Men Who Find Her Unappealing
Ms. Traditional	19%	41% ✚✚✚✚	23% ↓↓
Ms. Shy	8%	10% ✚	27% ↓↓↓
Ms. Smart	13%	34% ✚✚✚	16% ↓↓
Ms. Faithful	11%	27% ✚✚✚	13% ↓
Ms. Adventure	4%	51% ✚✚✚✚✚	18% ↓↓
Ms. Rebel	4%	38% ✚✚✚✚	27% ↓↓↓
Ms. Grounded	19%	30% ✚✚✚	12% ↓
Ms. Nice	22%	57% ✚✚✚✚✚✚	3%

✚ and ↓ = Approximately 10%

Figure 2: Proportion of Men with Each Public Persona and Their Popularity

	% of Men	Women Who Find Him Attractive	Women Who Find Him Unappealing
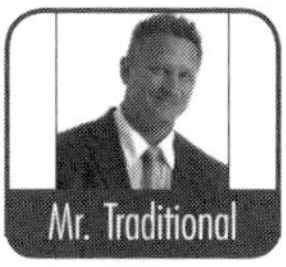 Mr. Traditional	14%	37% ✚✚✚✚	27% ↓↓↓
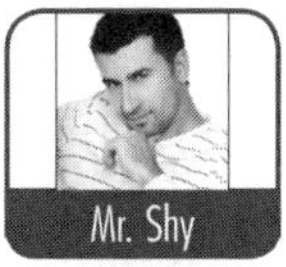 Mr. Shy	9%	6% ✚	38% ↓↓↓↓
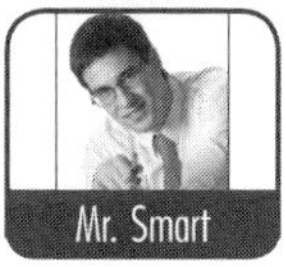 Mr. Smart	20%	31% ✚✚✚	30% ↓↓↓
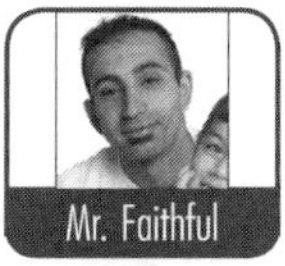 Mr. Faithful	14%	46% ✚✚✚✚✚	17% ↓↓
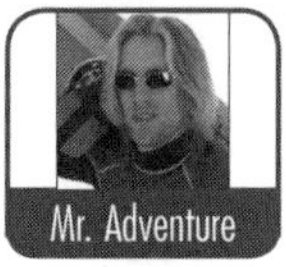 Mr. Adventure	5%	42% ✚✚✚✚	28% ↓↓↓
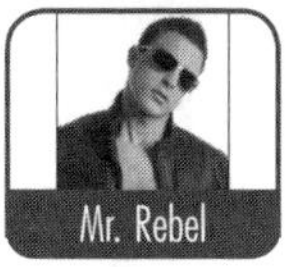 Mr. Rebel	5%	17% ✚✚	49% ↓↓↓↓↓
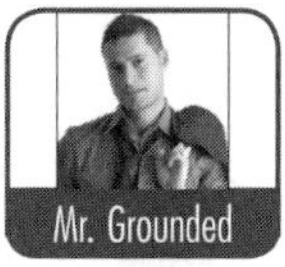 Mr. Grounded	11%	31% ✚✚✚	13% ↓
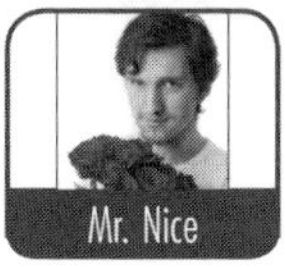 Mr. Nice	22%	67% ✚✚✚✚✚✚✚	3%

✚ and ↓ = Approximately 10%

Mr. Shy attractive, and about one in three women find this type unappealing. Ms. Shy fares a little better than Mr. Shy in popularity, but still only one in ten men find the shy type attractive.

The popularity of the other six types falls somewhere between these two extremes. In this way, most of the personas are quirky. They each have a core audience who appreciates their unique appeal. No persona is universally liked, and none is universally rejected.

After the Nice persona, the next most popular personas are the Traditional and Adventure types. Both are popular with about half of all men and women. The Traditional persona prompts polarized reactions: it is very popular with some but strongly disliked by others. Approximately one in three adults view this type as unappealing.

The next tier of popularity includes the Smart, Faithful, and Grounded personas. If your personality fits one of these personas, you can expect about one in three adults will find you very or extremely attractive. On the other extreme, about one in five will definitely not be attracted to your type.

Last but not least is the Rebel persona. This persona provokes both strong positive and negative reactions. Men tend to find Rebels more appealing than do women. About 40 percent of men say they find women who are Rebels attractive. In contrast, only about one in seven women say they are attracted to the Rebel type, and half of all women view Mr. Rebel as very or extremely unattractive.

The popularity of each public persona only tells part of the story, since your prospects as a single person are always a function of supply and demand. Take the Adventure type. This is a relatively rare type, but it's extremely popular. If you threw a party and invited one hundred men and one hundred women, there would be about four Ms. Adventures and fifty-one potential male suitors who like her type. That's twelve suitors per woman. Those are pretty good odds. There would be five Mr. Adventures at the party, and they would also have a great chance of meeting someone who's drawn to their personality, with at least eight female suitors per person.

When you look at it this way, the Traditional, Faithful, Nice, and Rebel personas all have a good chance of meeting someone who likes their personality type. For each of these personas, there are at least three times as many potential suitors as there are candidates with that type. Even Mr. Rebel, who is not especially popular, can expect to meet several women who will like his personality type.

Judging a Book by Its Cover

Is Personality Linked to Sexual Interests?

There's no substitute for talking openly and honestly with your partner about your sexual interests. But we all know these conversations are awkward and easy to put off.

Life would be a lot easier if there were a way to anticipate the sex drive and sexual interests of potential dates before you invest a lot of time in dating them. There's no perfect way to judge a book by its cover. However, it turns out that men and women's public personalities tend to offer fairly reliable clues about their sexual drive and interests.

Looking at the eight public personas we just reviewed, how many of these personality types have you dated? Have you noticed whether people with certain personality traits tended to be more interested in sex and sexual variety than others?

Take a look at Figure 3 (for women) and Figure 4 (for men). For each of the eight public personas, I've listed the proportion of men and women with high or very high sex drives and the proportion with Adventurous or Kinky sexual tastes. What immediately jumps out at you is that the personality types are divided into two sexual tiers.

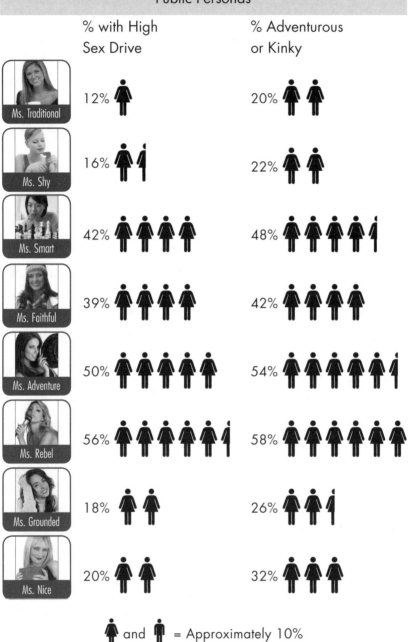

Figure 3: Sex Drive and Adventurousness of Women's Public Personas

% with High Sex Drive

% Adventurous or Kinky

Ms. Traditional — 12% — 20%

Ms. Shy — 16% — 22%

Ms. Smart — 42% — 48%

Ms. Faithful — 39% — 42%

Ms. Adventure — 50% — 54%

Ms. Rebel — 56% — 58%

Ms. Grounded — 18% — 26%

Ms. Nice — 20% — 32%

and = Approximately 10%

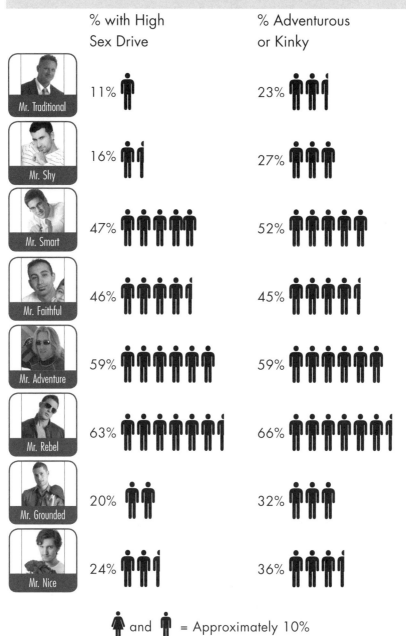

Figure 4: Sex Drive and Adventurousness of Men's Public Personas

There are four public personas with relatively few men and women with high sex drives or adventurous tastes. Only about one in five people with Traditional, Shy, Nice, or Grounded personality types have high sex drives. Only one in four has Adventurous or Kinky sexual tastes. So the vast majority of men and women in these persona groups have low or moderate sex drives and Vanilla or Mainstream sexual tastes.

So if you are looking to have a Mainstream sex life, your odds are very good that you can find a good match with this bunch. However, if you have a high sex drive and need a lot of sexual variety, you should probably be looking for one of the personality types in this next group.

People in the Smart, Faithful, Adventure, or Rebel groups are much more likely to have strong sexual interests. Roughly half of the men and women with these personality types have high or very high sex drives. About half also have Adventurous or Kinky sexual tastes.

Among the men in Figure 4, the differences are especially striking. If you meet either Mr. Rebel or Mr. Adventure, there's a two-out-of-three chance that he will have a high sex drive and be sexually adventurous.

Why Is It Hard to Match Couples Based on Both Personality and Sexual Interests?

The four personas we identified as the *least* sexual (Traditional, Shy, Nice, and Grounded) are among the most common and more popular personality types. If you have a low or moderate sex drive and Mainstream sexual tastes, this is good news, since you probably already like these types and there are lots of them out there to choose from.

However, if you have a high sex drive and adventurous tastes, the fact that there are lots of likable personality types out there that aren't very sexual is not good news. It also makes my job as a matchmaker very difficult and frustrating.

To illustrate some of the challenges, let's look at a sample case.

Betty is a forty-year-old single woman with a high sex drive and adventurous sexual tastes. Betty tells us she is tired of meeting sexual duds and wants to meet a sexual wild man.

The best strategy for finding a good sexual match for Betty is to pair her with Mr. Rebel. At least two out of three Rebels have high sex drives and are sexually adventurous. However, he's one of the least popular personas among women. There's only a one-in-seven chance that Betty will like his public personality. In fact, there's a fifty-fifty chance that Betty will find his personality very or extremely *un*attractive.

Another option is to match Betty with Mr. Adventure, since most of the men with this personality type have high sex drives and are sexually adventurous. Mr. Adventure also tends to be more popular than Mr. Rebel. About 40 percent of women find this personality type attractive, and only one in three find this type unattractive.

What if, instead of focusing on sex, Betty decides she is primarily interested in finding a husband with an appealing personality? Our best strategy is to match her with Mr. Nice. We know that two out of three women are very or extremely attracted to Mr. Nice, and almost none of them find him unappealing. Of course, the downside is that once Betty gets around to having sex with him, there's only a one-in-three chance that they will like to do the same things sexually, and there's only a one-in-four chance that he will want to have sex as often as she does.

The story is about the same if we match her with Mr. Faithful, which is the second most popular personality type. This brings us back to the third most popular type: Mr. Adventure. Of the available options, he is the most likely to be *both* a good personality match (42 percent chance) and a good sexual match (about 50 percent).

I hope your prospects are easier than Betty's. But if you're looking for a strong sexual connection with someone, you're probably going to have to weigh the relative importance of finding compatibility in the bedroom versus compatibility outside the bedroom.

Why Do Extroverted People Have More Sex?

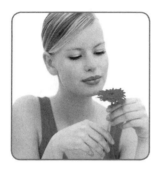 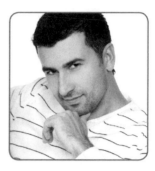

Ms. Shy   Mr. Shy

If you're trying to anticipate how sexual someone is going to be, one of the most important traits to watch for is *extroversion* or the extent to which someone is outgoing, social, active, and assertive. People who are extroverted report having a lot more sexual partners than introverted people, and they tend to have sex a lot more often.

Part of this may be due to opportunity. Extroverted personality types like Mr. and Ms. Adventure tend to have more friends. They meet more people and go to more parties than introverts, which gives them more opportunities to meet potential sexual partners.

Extroverts tend to be energized by social situations, while introverts like Mr. or Ms. Shy tend to find social interactions draining. So even if introverts enjoy sex as much as extroverts, they tend to find the process of seeking out sex and being social a lot more emotionally and physically draining.

The old adage "still waters run deep" can definitely be true. You may discover that Mr. or Ms. Shy is a sexual dynamo once the two of you finally connect. However, my studies suggest that this is the exception rather than the rule.

Can Dependability and Reliability Box You in Sexually?

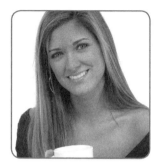 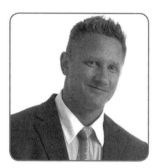

Ms. Traditional   Mr. Traditional

Another trait to keep an eye out for is *conscientiousness,* or the extent to which someone is organized, reliable, and efficient. These are all great qualities, but when it comes to sex, there may be a downside to dependability. People who are high in conscientiousness like Mr. or Ms. Traditional tend to be less interested in sex than their peers.[14] They tend to embrace structure, rules, and routines in life. This can make for a very safe and stable relationship, but it may not leave much room for sexual exploration or variety.

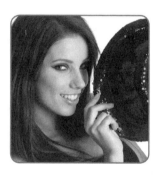 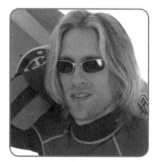

Ms. Adventure   Mr. Adventure

In contrast, people who tend to be more spontaneous and less structured in their work and social lives, like Mr. or Ms. Adventure, tend to be more spontaneous when it comes to sex as well. They tend to have sex earlier in a relationship, have sex more often, and are more interested in sexual variety than their more conservative peers.[15]

Is Smart Sexy?

Smart and creative people tend to be more sexual than people with few intellectual or artistic interests. Intellectual *openness* or the extent to which someone is curious, imaginative, and tolerant of new ideas is closely linked with sex drive and sexual adventurousness. People like Mr. and Ms. Smart tend to have sex more often and with more variety than people with more cautious, conservative, and pragmatic personalities.

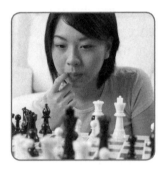 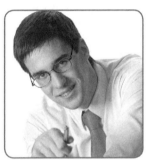

Ms. Smart   Mr. Smart

In my studies, men and women who described themselves as smart, intelligent, logical, and imaginative reported thinking about sex, fantasizing about sex, and having sex more often than people who did not see themselves as smart or intellectual. They also usually had a wider scope of sexual experiences, including experience with role-playing and other Kinky activities.[16]

Is There a Sexual Downside to Being Nice?

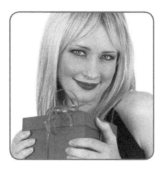

Ms. Nice

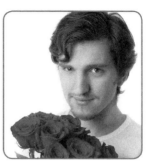

Mr. Nice

I was surprised the first time I saw the results in Figures 3 and 4 and saw how low Mr. and Ms. Nice fell in the ranking of sex drives and adventurousness. It didn't make sense to me that these kind and accommodating men and women would be the least interested in sex and sexual exploration. They are warm, generous, trusting, and compassionate. What's not to love? Aren't these sexually appealing qualities?

But there's something about these personality traits that appears to get in the way of sexual expression. It turns out that one of the things that sets this group apart is their approach to sex and love. They are more likely than any other persona group to view sex as an expression of love and emotional intimacy.

They also tend to be much less casual about sex. While Mr. and Ms. Nice are single, they tend to wait longer to have sex and have sex less often while they're dating. Most say they want to have a strong emotional connection with someone before they have sex.

Even after they're in a relationship, Mr. and Ms. Nice still have sex less often than people with other personality types. They are more interested in making love than just having sex. They are turned on by romance and emotional closeness. Unfortunately, long-term relationships do not always accommodate this approach to sex. Kids, finances, and busy schedules tend to undermine romance and romantic sex.

Mr. and Ms. Nice also hate conflict and hurt feelings. While some couples can argue and then have great make-up sex, conflict is a total turnoff to Mr. and Ms. Nice. Since all couples have fights, you may end up waiting a long time for a perfect peaceful connection.

Mr. and Ms. Nice tend to be sexually faithful. They are by far the least likely to cheat on their partners. They also tend to be more concerned with satisfying their partner sexually and set rather high standards for their sexual performance. All good things, right?

The downside to worrying about your partner's sexual satisfaction is that you can neglect your own sexual wishes. Indeed, Mr. and Ms. Nice are less likely than those in other groups to initiate sex or ask for what they want sexually. They are also less likely to have sexual fantasies, in part because, unlike other groups, they almost never fantasize about someone other than their partner.

Is There a Sexual Upside to Being a Jerk?

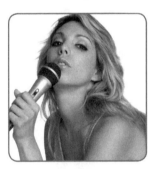
Ms. Rebel

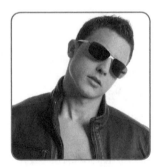
Mr. Rebel

The two most sexual personality types also happen to be the two groups who are the least concerned with being nice, kind, and accommodating. People with the Rebel or Adventure personality types tend to be guarded, stubborn, and shrewd. They are also the most likely to have high sex drives and adventurous sexual tastes.

Rebels and Adventurers tend to be straightforward and assertive about *whom* they want and *what* they want sexually. They are persistent and willing to take risks. A man with these qualities, for example, is the type of guy who will go up to a woman he finds attractive and introduce himself, even though he knows she might blow him off or roll her eyes at him.

They are tough-skinned and not crushed by rejection, like Mr. or Ms. Nice might be. They also don't worry about hurting other people's feelings. They don't go out on pity dates or have pity sex.

Rebels and Adventurers also know how to be selfish sexually. They are more likely than any other group to initiate sex, even if they are unsure whether their partner is interested. They are also the *least* concerned about sexual performance. They are not afraid to tell their lovers what they want and how they want it.

Where Are You Willing to Make Compromises?

Compatibility always involves trade-offs. You might be able to find everything you're looking for in one person. But you might also spend the rest of your life looking for this perfect combination and never find it.

Life is a little easier for men and women with low or moderate sex drives and Mainstream sexual tastes. You're much more likely to find a sexually compatible partner among the personality types you already find attractive.

If you have a high sex drive and adventurous (or kinky) sexual tastes, you're probably going to have a tougher time finding a good match. As we've seen, the most popular, nicest, and most dependable personality types also tend to be the least sexual. If you like outgoing, rebellious, and spontaneous types, you have a better chance of finding a strong sexual connection than if you like shy, caring, and dependable types.

If you're looking for a partner with a relatively rare combination of personality and sexual interests, then at least you know what you're up against. If nothing else, I hope you can at least feel reassured that you're not imagining things. Searching for your ideal mate is challenging. You may have to make some trade-offs and decide which qualities are absolutely essential and which you can live without.

Chapter 4

Keeping the Spark Alive

Staying Attracted

What Obstacles Do You Face as a Couple?

If you're already married or in a committed relationship, finding a new lover that perfectly matches your sex drive and interests is not an option. So if you and your current partner have lost your sexual spark or seem to be mismatched on the basic dimensions of sexual compatibility, we need to focus on creating a sex life that can be satisfying to both of you.

Keeping the sexual spark alive in a long-term relationship is never easy. I have yet to meet a couple who did not struggle at some point (and often at multiple points) in their relationship with sexual boredom and loss of sexual interest.

In this chapter we're going to look at two obstacles to keeping the sexual spark alive. The first is staying attracted to each other personally and physically. It's easy to take each other for granted and to stop noticing the qualities that once drew you together. We'll look at several things you can do to rekindle your attraction to your partner and keep him or her interested in you as well.

Then we'll look at several strategies for spicing up your sex life. We'll take the exercises from Chapter 2 and turn them into action plans for adding more variety to your sex life. We'll look at ways you can have affair sex without having an affair. We'll see why it's important to be proactive in spicing up your sex life *before* either of you is tempted to be unfaithful. But for those who find it difficult (or impossible) to stay monogamous, we'll look at two alternatives to traditional monogamous marriage.

How Can You Stay Attracted to Each Other?

There are many different types of attraction that can draw two people together. Fortunately, men and women find a wide variety of physical types to be attractive. As we saw in the last chapter, there are also a variety of personality types that men and women find appealing. I hope the exercises in the last chapter reminded you of some of the qualities that first drew you to your partner and why the two of you became a couple. Now, let's look at some of the challenges the two of you face in keeping that mutual attraction alive and fresh.

The first and most obvious challenge is that both of you are going to change physically as you get older, put on weight, have babies, or go through other physical changes. That cute face you kissed on your first date is not the same face looking back at you five years later, ten years later, or fifty years later. That body you lusted after when you first had sex is not the same body lying next to you tonight. Chances are it's bigger, flabbier, and less toned.

With all these changes, it's really miraculous to see how many couples stay attracted to each other. In my studies, about one in three couples say they are *more* physically attracted to each other now than when they first got together. In a moment, I'll share a few tips on sustaining your physical attraction.

In addition to all the external changes, we also tend to change and evolve internally. A lot of people complain that their partners used to talk and act in a particular way when they first met, but changed after they settled into a relationship.

The good news is that you both still have those personality traits inside you. You both have the potential to act that way again (joke around more often, be more spontaneous, show more compassion, and so forth). The challenge is restructuring your relationship dynamic so that these old behaviors are rewarded and maintained long term. Let's look at a few things you can do to share your best side with your partner and bring out his or her best side as well.

How Can You Stay Personally Appealing to Your Partner?

It's easy to fall into a rut in relationships and start playing predictable roles as a wife, husband, mother, or father. It's surprisingly easy to start reading from predictable relationship scripts and stop interacting as individuals.

Chances are you are both the same interesting and quirky individuals you were when you first met. But those individuals often get pushed aside due to work and family pressures. So it's important that the two of you get reacquainted and reintroduce yourselves to each other from time to time.

Regular date nights are a great way to do this. They give you a chance to talk about interesting things and silly things and just have fun, rather than focus all your interactions on the logistics of family life.

I recommend you put the same effort you used to put into dates with strangers into your dates with your partner. Back in your dating years, you probably made a special effort to highlight your best personality traits on dates. Try to do the same the next time you are on a date with your partner. Go back and take a look at the personality traits you picked as describing you in the last chapter. Which of these traits come naturally to you? When was the last time you shared this part of yourself with your partner?

When couples stop sharing their best side with their partner, they tend to blame their kids, their jobs, their finances, and so forth for getting them in this rut. It's tempting to want to fix all the other pressures and stressors in your life first, and *then* start changing how you interact with your partner. However, it's a trap (and a cop-out) to think that the only way you can improve your relationship is to make major life changes. Sometimes even a few small changes can make a big difference.

As a start, identify two or three traits that (1) you know your partner finds attractive and (2) you would like to bring out in yourself more often. Then find opportunities to bring this part of yourself out again. If you used to be imaginative and spontaneous, for example, find small ways you can share this part of yourself with your partner again.

Don't expect your partner to notice right away or appreciate the effort you put into it. It may take a little time for your partner to appreciate that you are sharing your best side again. Still, if these are personal qualities that you like about yourself anyway, then you can enjoy being the real you, regardless of who notices.

How Can You Bring Out the Best in Your Partner's Personality?

It's easier to change yourself and your behavior than to change your partner's behavior. Still, there are several things you can do to help bring out your partner's best side and see more of the personal qualities that once drew you to him or her.

First, you need to find ways to remind your partner that you still find him or her attractive. Everyone needs and values praise and compliments. Unfortunately, couples tend to stop noticing the good things about each other and often only comment on each other's shortcomings.

Look at the exercises in the last chapter and the public persona that best fits your partner. Pick out a few of his or her best traits. Then find an opportunity to let your partner know you still notice and admire these qualities. It can be as simple as saying, "It's been awhile since I told you, but I wanted you to know how much I still love the way you..." Remind your partner of the qualities you still admire, find endearing, and find sexy.

If you would like to see your partner show more of a particular quality or behavior, praise him or her whenever he or she does it. Complaining about it or asking your partner to be a particular way rarely works. Criticism usually just makes things worse.

So, instead, watch for a time when he or she does it (or does something close to it) and reward it in some way. It can be as simple as saying, "I love it when you..." or "Thank you for..." To really pour it on, you can give your partner a gift or do something he or she will appreciate as a way of reinforcing the behavior.

I don't advocate treating your partner like a pet, but we are all animals, and all animals learn through reward and reinforcement. Animal behaviorists teach lions to jump through hoops and coach dolphins to turn backflips by starting with activities the animals already do and then rewarding each progressive step toward the behavior they want to create. The challenge is finding a treat that your partner will see as a reward, and offering it at each step toward the change you want to create.

How Can I Make My Partner Feel More Attractive?

Dealing with changes in physical attraction can be a lot more complicated, but I believe the same basic principles apply. You need to remind yourself of the physical features and qualities you find attractive in your partner, and then let your partner know that you still find him or her sexy and physically attractive.

In my studies, couples who say they are satisfied with their sex lives tend to compliment their partners a lot and specifically comment on how sexy, beautiful, or handsome their partner looks. So my first bit of advice is to learn how to give good compliments.

As relationships mature, our compliments tend to get more general. Saying "I love you" usually becomes the standard way of expressing endearment. I have nothing against saying "I love you" and saying it often, but it's not a substitute for expressions of attraction or desire. So it's important to remind your partner that you still find him or her sexy and desirable.

All of us tie a lot of our self-image into how our face looks. So it's important to remind your partner that you still find his or her face appealing and attractive. Remind him that he's still handsome. Remind her that her face is as beautiful as the day you first met.

Incorporating a specific reference to the face can be awkward. If your partner is insecure, a compliment can even backfire (for example, "Are you saying you still like my face but think my body is fat?"). To avoid this sort of disaster, offer a broader compliment and fold in specific compliments about several things, including his or her face. You can also convey the same message by gently caressing your partner's face while you say how beautiful or handsome she or he is.

How Can I Continue to Feel Attractive?

Continuing to find your partner's face and body attractive as you age can be a challenge. But I think the bigger challenge (especially for women) is continuing to find yourself sexy and attractive. If you don't appreciate your own beauty and sex appeal, it's hard to believe that your partner finds you sexy, no matter how often he or she compliments you or reassures you.

It's hard to adjust to the changes you see in the mirror as you age. Aging is a moving target. Just when you start to adjust to how your face and body has changed, it changes again. Writer and director Nora Ephron made a great observation about this: "Anything you think is wrong with your body at the age of thirty-five you will be nostalgic for at the age of forty-five."[17]

I specialized in geriatrics during my clinical training, so I worked in a lot of nursing homes. I remember several patients telling me that the hardest thing about aging is *looking* old but *feeling* young. Now that I'm getting older myself, I've come to appreciate how frustrating this disconnect between the external you and the internal you truly is.

The morphology of how our faces age also works against us. As you age, your face sags, and the corners of your mouth tend to also sag. This can put a permanent scowl on your face. When I was young, my neutral facial expression looked pleasant and peaceful. Now, my neutral expression looks tired and sad. So I've been trying to smile more often. For a while, I was trying to keep a constant smile on my face, until I saw my reflection in a window and realized I looked like a lunatic.

There are medical options (like plastic surgery, Botox, or collagen) to try to slow or alter these facial changes. But these interventions can change your face in other ways as well.

There are no simple solutions. If you find one, please let me know.

One of my elderly patients once told me, "You have to make the future your friend." At the time, I had no idea what she meant, but I've recently started to appreciate her wisdom.

I think if you look in the mirror and only see what you've lost and see the future as your enemy, then you are bound to hate what you see. If you can appreciate where you are and look forward to where you are going, then your future is your friend. Perhaps then, that face in the mirror won't be so scary.

One practical thing you can do to help move your attitudes in this direction is to find good role models for aging gracefully. It is unfair and unrealistic to compare your face to individuals who are much younger or have millions to spend on plastic surgery. So you need to find role models with similar facial features who show it's possible to age naturally and continue to be beautiful (or handsome).

Don't waste your time looking for these in most magazines, since the models tend to fit a narrow idea of beauty and are airbrushed to look preternaturally perfect. You may have better luck looking to actors in television or movies, which are a little more diverse than they used to be. Maybe you can find a role model among your friends or family. Regardless, find one person or several people who can remind you that it's possible to look sexy and feel sexy at any age.

Spicing Up Your Sex Life

How Can You Spice Up Your Sex Life?

It's hard to know going into a relationship whether you and your partner are going to be satisfied with your sexual routine five, ten, or twenty years later. So try not to blame yourself or your partner if you arrive at a point in your relationship where you long for a little more sexual variety.

The first step is to make sure that both of you accept responsibility for improving your sex life. It's time to set aside blame for how you got into the rut. Focus instead on working together to get out of it. It's also important to recognize that it will take time, energy, and some trial-and-error experimentation to spice up your sex life. Not everything you try will work. You will get frustrated and discouraged. So you have to enter into this process with patience and a sense of humor.

Oftentimes, the dissatisfied partner has no suggestions for what the two of you should try out or do differently. He or she is sort of like a kid in the middle of summer break who mopes around saying, "I'm bored," and expects you to fix it. Although both partners have to work together to improve the situation, the reality is that if *you* are dissatisfied, *you* have to be willing to take the lead and make suggestions about what to do and try.

I recommend you *both* complete the first two exercises in Chapter 2. The first one asks you to identify the sexual activities that you have tried and the ones you would like to try in the future. The second exercise focuses specifically on Kinky sexual interests. I suggest buying *two* copies of this book, but if that is not feasible, I suppose photocopying the exercises is okay too. Based on these exercises, each of you should prepare separately the following three lists:

✓✓ *More Please:* These are sexual activities that you've enjoyed in the past and want to continue to enjoy in the future. Some of these are part of your sexual routine. However, there may be other items on the list that you both enjoyed but failed to incorporate into your regular routine.

One mistake that couples make is to assume they have to try lots of new activities in order to spice up their sex life. Sometimes the fastest and easiest solution is to retry several activities that you've enjoyed before but stopped doing or overlooked for whatever reason.

Another similar strategy is to take activities you both currently enjoy, but do them in a different way, in a different location, or in a different order from what you are used to. Sometimes it can take surprisingly little to break old habits and make something old seem like something new.

✗✓ *Would Most Like to Explore:* These are sexual activities you have not tried but are interested in trying. Compare which items fit in this category for both you and your partner. Obviously, any activities that you both want to try are great candidates for your sexual experiments.

✗? *Most Curious About:* These are activities you have not tried but are curious about. Compare the items on this list with the items on the previous list. If one of you is definitely interested in exploring an activity, and the other is curious about it, then you can at least talk about it as a possibility.

Remember that pressuring and begging rarely work. If your partner is curious about something you are interested in trying, ask questions like: What about this do you find interesting or exciting? What do you think you would enjoy about it? The more excited your partner is about the idea, the more likely he or she will be willing to give it a try.

Then ask questions about what your partner is afraid of or uncomfortable with: What are you afraid might happen if we try it? What can I do to make you more comfortable with trying this?

You'll hopefully find some additional inspiration later in Part 3 when we explore the different components of sexual chemistry. I recommend you pay special attention to the sections on sexual role-play in Part 3 and in Chapter 12, since exploring each other's sexual fantasies through role-play can be a great way to spice up your sex life. Still, it never hurts to start with the basics and expand what you do sexually and when and how you have sex before you tackle more advanced sexual dynamics like role-play.

Finally, talk about and pick someone who is going to take the lead when you have sex. All complicated interpersonal activities, whether it's dancing, mountain climbing, or adventurous sex, work best when someone takes the lead and serves as the guide. Couples with more egalitarian sex roles tend to be somewhat less sexually adventurous than couples with a partner who takes the lead sexually. So when the two of you embark on a night of sexual experimentation, decide who is going to take the lead. Ideally, the two of you can take turns and switch off the role of sexual guide on different nights.

How Are You Going to Stay Monogamous?

Staying monogamous is easy for some couples and really difficult (or impossible) for others. I encourage single people to think long and hard about their interest and capacity for monogamy *before* they get married or commit to a monogamous relationship. But if you're already in a relationship, it's probably too late for that.

If you've made a monogamous commitment, then you need to have a plan for *how* you are going to stay monogamous. The biggest threat to monogamy for most couples is sexual boredom.

As we discussed in Chapter 2, there are very real psychological and physiological reasons for why we tend to habituate to certain types of arousal when we have the same experiences over and over again. What is initially new and exciting tends to become predictable and boring. Madame Bovary—one of the great sexual heroines in literature—put it this way: "And the charm of novelty, gradually slipping away like a garment, laid bare the eternal monotony of passion, whose forms and phrases are forever the same."[18]

If you know going into a relationship that you really enjoy the novelty of sex with different partners, then you have to replace one form of novelty and variety with another form. You have to make sex with the same partner *seem* like having sex with multiple partners. As we'll see in Part 3, one way to accomplish this is through sexual role-play. By pretending to be different people, you can trick your mind and body into experiencing each other in new ways.

How Can You Have Affair Sex without Having an Affair?

Another approach to maintaining sexual novelty is to try to have affair sex without having an affair. There's a reason why affair sex is so arousing. The newness of your partner's body, being rushed, meeting in a secret place, and so forth interact to change the sexual who, what, where, when, and how of the experience. So the more you can mix up the location and timing of sex with your partner, the more you can mimic the excitement and novelty of a sexual affair.

I believe it's crucial to be proactive and work hard at making monogamy fun. It's unfortunate, but most couples refuse to put much effort into their sex lives until something goes wrong. They wait until one of them has an affair, or at least thinks about having an affair, before they're willing to put some effort and imagination into their sex life.

The downside to this reactive approach is that by the time one of you has an affair or threatens to have an affair, a lot of anger and resentment gets mixed into the relationship. By that point, you not only have to deal with sexual issues but emotional and trust issues as well.[19] Why not skip that phase and spice up your sex life before you betray and hurt each other?!

So I encourage you to meet your partner at a cheap motel. Strip off each other's clothes. Skip things you normally do and try new things. If you are usually tender, be rough. Mix things up and trick your bodies into feeling like they're having sex with new and exciting partners.

What If You Don't Want to Be Monogamous?

I am not here to make judgments or prescribe codes of conduct. You bought my book, and I love you for it. Still, I believe that if you make a monogamous commitment to someone, you should honor it. If you know you cannot honor it (for whatever reason), then you need to tell your partner how you feel.

Monogamy isn't for everyone. So it's worth at least discussing some alternative nontraditional approaches to structuring your relationship. One option is to have sex with a third person or another couple for a one-time fling or an ongoing thing. Another alternative is to create an open relationship so you can each pursue your sexual interests separately, without lying to each other or pretending to be someone you're not. Let's look at each of these options in more detail.

How Do You Approach a Three-Way or Four-Way?

Most everyone has fantasized about threesomes, group sex, or swinging with another couple, but few make this a reality. These are among the most complicated sexual adventures you can embark on.

They only work if *everyone* has excellent self-esteem, has good communication skills, and is not prone to jealousy. That rules out most of us.

You should also keep in mind that the reality of threesomes or group sex can be different from your fantasies. Going in this direction can be a big mistake if your relationship is unstable. If the two of you are not connected sexually, adding a third (or fourth) person is only going to exaggerate these differences.

It's also not something that tends to work spontaneously or with a "let's see what happens" attitude. Everyone needs to talk up front about their expectations and agree about safety and limits.

With that said, let's look at three approaches to inviting someone else into your sexual relationship. The best approach for you and your partner would depend on your goals, comfort level, and what turns you on.

With the first approach, there are three participants, but only two are playing at any one time. This allows the third person to watch and give the other two an audience. If you're a voyeur, maybe you would be turned on by watching your partner having sex with someone else. If you're more of an exhibitionist, maybe you would enjoy having a stranger watch you and your partner have sex or like the idea of having your partner watch you having sex with someone else.

A good way to test the waters and explore whether watching or being watched would be a turn-on (or a turnoff) is to have sex in front of a mirror. You might also consider videotaping sex or try webcam sex to see if you're both truly ready to add a third.

With the second approach, everyone plays together. You play with the new person, your partner plays with the new person, you all play simultaneous, and so forth. It's important to talk up-front about comfort zones, preferences, and limits. This is not a good time for "don't ask, don't tell." It is also important that everyone stay involved and no one is left feeling like a third wheel.

The third approach is to turn the three-way into a four-way. Having two couples often reduces the risk that one person is left out or that a couple feels threatened by an outsider. If this is your thing, there are a number of swingers groups, parties, and websites to choose from.

Great sex between two people rarely just happens, and the more players you add to the equation, the more assumptions and misunderstandings can get in the way. With that said, you may find "the more, the merrier." It may be something you try once and never want to do again, or it could be a way to have sex with other partners while still maintaining your sexual commitment to each other.

Would an Open Relationship Work?

Individuals in open relationships have an explicit arrangement with their primary partner that allows them to have sex with other people. The most common example is an open marriage, where both spouses are free to have sex outside their relationship. For some couples, these outside sexual pursuits supplement their existing sexual relationship. It's like a sexual dessert on top of your regular sexual diet at home.

For other couples, whose sex lives have fizzled or disappeared, outside sexual pursuits become their primary sexual outlet. This can work for couples who still love each other deeply and remain committed to staying together, but recognize that they are not going to be able to meet each other's sexual needs.

The explicit arrangement can be in the form of "don't ask, don't tell." Or it can involve a detailed set of rules (not in our bed, no kissing, no more than once a year, always tell me, never tell me, etc.).

Open relationships remain a taboo topic in our culture. Folks who go down this road often find themselves in uncharted territory. It's certainly not a good strategy for individuals who are poor communicators or prone to jealously. Again, that rules out most of us. But if you want to stay together and can commit to being honest and patient with each other and with the outside partners you'll connect with along the way, then maybe you can be a sexual pioneer and find a way to make a nontraditional arrangement work.

PART 3

Secrets of Sexual Chemistry

Chapter 5

The Three Ingredients of Sexual Chemistry

Great Sex

Is It What You Do or How You Do It?

What is the best sex you've ever had? If you can't narrow it down to one absolute best, think about your top five sexual encounters. What made them special? What set these magical experiences apart from one another? What set them apart from more mediocre encounters?

Who is the best sexual partner you've ever had? What made him or her such a great lover? I bet he or she probably wasn't the most physically attractive person you've been with. A gorgeous face or a killer body rarely guarantees a hot sexual connection. As a matter of fact, it's often folks with average looks who turn out to be sexual rock stars.

What Makes Great Sex Great?

So, what makes great sex great? The particular combination of sexual activities obviously plays a part. That's why Parts 1 and 2 focused on how to find (or create) a sexual connection with a partner who has similar levels of sex drive and sexual adventurousness. Still, *what* you do sexually isn't the key ingredient to great sex. I'm sure you've enjoyed the exact same sexual menu with different lovers and felt very different levels of sexual joy and satisfaction.

What makes great sex great is primarily about *how* you have sex. It's about how your sexual style meshes (or clashes) with your partner's style.

That's the focus of Part 3. We'll explore the factors that go into creating sexual chemistry. Specifically, we'll look at three core ingredients (emotion, power, and intensity) that can combine to create hot sex. You'll learn about your own personal recipe for great sex and which combination of ingredients works best for you.

Sexual chemistry is different from sexual compatibility. Chemistry is something you create in the moment as part of your sexual connection with someone. You can see chemistry at work (or its absence) in a single sexual encounter. Compatibility centers on the long-term fit between the needs, desires, and interests of a couple. In Parts 1 and 2, we made some progress in defining the basic components of sexual compatibility. But having similar sex drives and a need for variety is usually not enough for long-term compatibility. A great sex life requires a sexual spark. It requires chemistry. So now we are going to explore what this means for you and the type of connection you are searching for. We will see how the basic ingredients of sexual chemistry come together in a single encounter and how (if you're lucky) you can find a partner who can re-create this formula again and again over the long haul.

Why Should We Explore Your Inner Sex Life?

Most of the book so far has focused on relationships and different types and varieties of sexual activity. In Part 3 we're going to broaden our scope to include your *inner* sex life—your sexual thoughts and fantasies—that runs alongside and often independently of your external sex life.

Why should we focus more on your inner sex life? First, your inner sex life plays a big role in your enjoyment of sex over your lifetime. If we add up all the sexual sensations and experiences you will ever have, chances are at least half or more of them occur internally, in your thoughts and fantasies.[20] Interpersonal sex is great, but these experiences can be few and far between. You've probably gone through periods in the past, and may go through times in the future, when your sexual fantasies serve as your primary or only sexual outlet.[21]

The second reason to explore your inner sex life is because it interconnects with your external sex life in interesting and influential ways. I've listed some of the interconnections in Figure 1.[22] Our current and past sexual partners and our most memorable sexual experiences obviously play a big role in shaping our sexual fantasies and daydreams. Women tend to fantasize less than men, and most women say they fantasize about their *current* husband or boyfriend. Men are much more likely to fantasize about previous partners, potential lovers, or desired but unobtainable lovers (such as celebrities).

Our inner sex lives also shape who we find sexually attractive and the kinds of sexual experiences we seek out. Whether they're aware of it or not, a lot of single men and women approach sex and dating like a producer putting on a theatrical play. You have a script for what you would like to happen, and you set out to cast the part of your ideal lover with a certain type in mind. So to understand who you find sexually attractive and why you approach sex with particular likes and dislikes, we'll need to explore your fantasy lovers, settings, and roles.

Figure 1: How Do Your Internal and External Sex Lives Influence Each Other?

→ Create a sexual experience inspired by fantasy
→ Seduce a sexual partner who fits a fantasy
→ Incorporate fantasies into sexual role-play
→ Fantasize about another partner while having sex

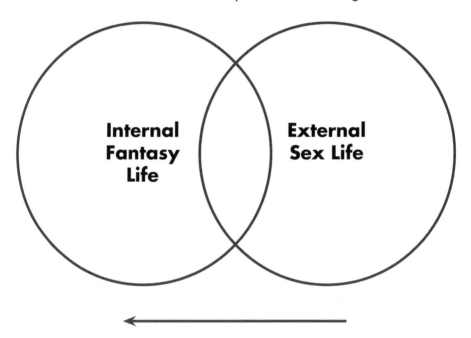

Internal Fantasy Life

External Sex Life

← Fantasize about current or former partner(s)
← Fantasize about possible future lovers
← Fantasize about previous sexual experiences
← Fantasize about anticipated sexual encounters

How Can We Describe Sexual Chemistry?

Sexual chemistry is sort of like the weather. It's obvious when it runs hot or cold, but it's difficult to predict and full of surprises. Everybody talks about it and has opinions about it, but nobody does anything about it.

A few years ago I decided to take a close look at what people describe as sexual chemistry. I asked hundreds of men and women to describe the best sex they ever had. I also asked them to describe encounters that were sexually disappointing or times when the chemistry was obviously off.

What I discovered was that similar themes popped up again and again. People talked about times when the sexual energy clicked, when they were on the same emotional wavelength. For some men and women, great sex was slow and tender, while others loved it fast and intense. Issues of power, taking charge, and surrender came up again and again.

After a while I realized that I had seen these core themes at play before. As Yogi Berra put it, it was "like déjà vu all over again."

It turns out that I had studied the perfect framework for studying sexual chemistry twenty years ago in graduate school. It's called *symbolic interactionism*.[23] In a nutshell, this school of thought argues that every person, place, activity, and thing has both an *objective* reality and a *symbolic* meaning. Every person, object, and situation provokes an emotional reaction and can be expected to behave in a particular way. An amusement park is good and fun. A prison is bad and dangerous. A car can move quickly, a tree can sway, and rocks tend to stay in place.

As an individual, I'm sure you have your own unique view of the world. Nevertheless, you also share a common culture and language with the people in your life. Sociologists add that on a deeper level you also share a common *symbolic framework* for what everyone and everything means.

This framework consists of three core dimensions:

- *Negative to Positive Emotion:* This is the overall emotional tone associated with an object or activity. We tend to view the world on a continuum from bad to good. Things tend to provoke negative emotions (unhappy, sad, annoyed, unsatisfied) or positive emotions (happy, joyous, pleased, satisfied).

- *Weak to Strong Power:* We associate a certain level of power with different jobs, objects, and activities. They can be rated on a continuum from weak (fragile, vulnerable, submissive, unimportant) to strong (potent, powerful, dominant, influential).

- *Slow to Fast Activity:* This is the actual or potential movement associated with a person, place, or pursuit. It's represented on a continuum from slow (relaxed, calm, stable, inactive) to fast (aroused, excited, changing, active).

I have to admit I struggled with this framework for years. It was too simple (or elegant) for my tiny mind to comprehend.

"How can a toaster have an activity level?" I asked at one seminar. "My toaster doesn't make me feel happy *or* sad."

The sociologists around the conference table tried to explain that these were meanings that our culture and language *invest* in objects, not qualities of the object itself.

"Which is faster: a toaster or a rock?" one of the grad students threw at me impatiently. It was obvious she thought I was dumber than both.[24]

I don't recall how that exchange ended. But twenty years later, I have a renewed appreciation for these basic dimensions and for being able to describe people, places, and actions with a simple, common vocabulary. In fact, we are going to explore how the three dimensions of emotion, power, and activity serve as the core ingredients that make up sexual chemistry.

How Would You Describe Your Ideal Sexual Experience?

Take a moment to complete Exercise 1. Think of the best sex you've ever had or your favorite sexual fantasy. Specifically, ask yourself these questions:

- Who's your ideal or fantasy lover?
- Where's the ideal place or setting for sex?
- What role do you like to play sexually?
- What role would you like your ideal partner to play?

Then use the rating bars to describe each of these elements in terms of their emotional tone, power, and activity level.

Where Do We Go from Here?

I realize that boiling down your favorite sexual memories or fantasies into a handful of ratings is a little weird. What we're hoping to do is discover the themes that pop up in how you approach sex.

If you had a hard time making the ratings, don't worry. In the next three chapters we'll take a closer look at each of the three ingredients to sexual chemistry. These are brief chapters meant to clarify the specific factors that turn you on or off. In Chapter 6 we'll explore whether you're drawn to sex that is light and wholesome or dark and dirty. In Chapter 7 we'll look at how dominance, submission, and other exchanges of power can enhance (or undermine) your enjoyment of sex. Then, in Chapter 8, we'll compare men and women who approach sex as a fast and intense experience filled with excitement, change, and movement versus those who approach sex as a slow and tender journey that is relaxing, sensual, and focused.

This will set the stage for us to look at how these different ingredients combine to create unique sexual styles. In Chapter 9 we'll explore how your sexual style expresses itself in your inner sex life. We'll discover which of the eight fantasy zones you find most exciting and intriguing, as well as the zones that make you feel uncomfortable.

Exercise 1: Describe Your Ideal Sexual Experience

Put an X on the point along each continuum which describes your fantasy lover, setting, and sexual activity.

How would you describe <u>your ideal lover?</u>

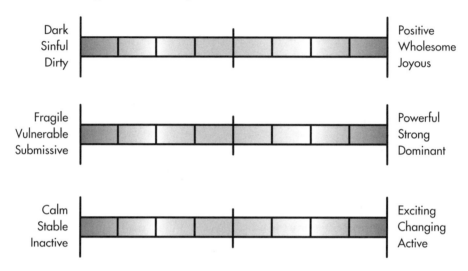

Dark Sinful Dirty		Positive Wholesome Joyous
Fragile Vulnerable Submissive		Powerful Strong Dominant
Calm Stable Inactive		Exciting Changing Active

How would you describe the ideal <u>setting or location</u> for sex?

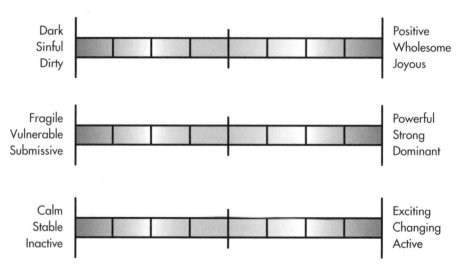

Dark Sinful Dirty		Positive Wholesome Joyous
Fragile Vulnerable Submissive		Powerful Strong Dominant
Calm Stable Inactive		Exciting Changing Active

Exercise 1 (continued)

How would you describe <u>your ideal sexual role</u> or sexual actions?

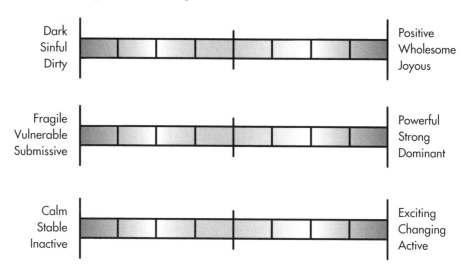

Dark / Sinful / Dirty — Positive / Wholesome / Joyous

Fragile / Vulnerable / Submissive — Powerful / Strong / Dominant

Calm / Stable / Inactive — Exciting / Changing / Active

How would you describe <u>your partner's role</u> or sexual actions?

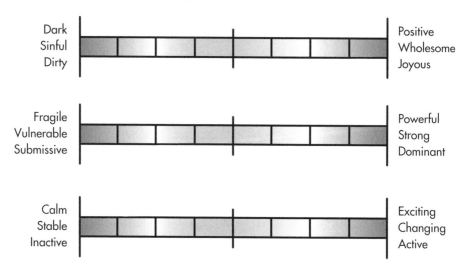

Dark / Sinful / Dirty — Positive / Wholesome / Joyous

Fragile / Vulnerable / Submissive — Powerful / Strong / Dominant

Calm / Stable / Inactive — Exciting / Changing / Active

You'll see how your desires, fears, and insecurities interact to push you toward certain fantasy zones and away from others.

Finally, in Chapter 10, we'll explore how your preferences for specific mixtures of emotion, power, and intensity can combine to create a personal sexual style or sexual personality that only comes out when you express yourself sexually. Your sexual persona may be aligned and consistent with your public persona, or it could be a distinct and separate part of who you are. We'll see which sexual styles tend to mesh and create sexual fireworks and which ones tend to clash and sink relationships.

Great sexual chemistry occurs when all three dimensions—emotion, power, and activity—mesh together. Most men and women are turned on by partners with *similar* emotion and activity styles and *contrasting* power styles. A woman with a slow, sensual, and wholesome approach to sex who likes to play a more passive sexual role will have the best sexual chemistry with a man who also likes sensual and wholesome sex and is comfortable taking the lead sexually.

As we'll see, this is only one of sixty-four possible combinations of sexual styles. There are many possible configurations of sexual likes and dislikes and many possible ways men and women's styles can fit or clash. When you think of all the ways things can mismatch, it's sort of surprising that couples ever click sexually. Fortunately, however, there are a variety of ways that couples can adapt to and adjust to each other's sexual styles.

Learning the secrets to sexual chemistry in Part 3 will set the stage for learning how to find a partner with whom you can share great chemistry (Chapter 11) or reignite your sexual spark with your existing partner (Chapter 12). We'll look at ways you can enhance your inner and external sex life by embracing your sexual style and preferences. We'll look at strategies for finding a partner with a compatible sexual style and what you can do to improve your connection if your styles don't automatically click.

Chapter 6

Emotions and Sex

Do You Enjoy the Lighter or Darker Side of Sex?

Emotional Style

Which Emotional Style Is Sexier?

Are you turned on by sex that is naughty or nice? Are you drawn to lovers who are wholesome and innocent or dangerous and sinful?

Each person brings his or her own unique emotions and expectations to sex. Some people prefer sex that is pure, safe, and kind. But others find this boring and uninteresting. They're drawn to sex that is primitive, wicked, and edgy.

It's amazing that sex can express itself in so many different ways and provoke completely opposite reactions in people. To see where your interests fall, let's explore the type of qualities you find sexiest in a lover. If you're attracted to women, try Exercise 1. If you're attracted to men, try Exercise 2.

There are six pairs of options in two columns. Pick the option that you find sexier. Are you drawn to partners who are nice or naughty?

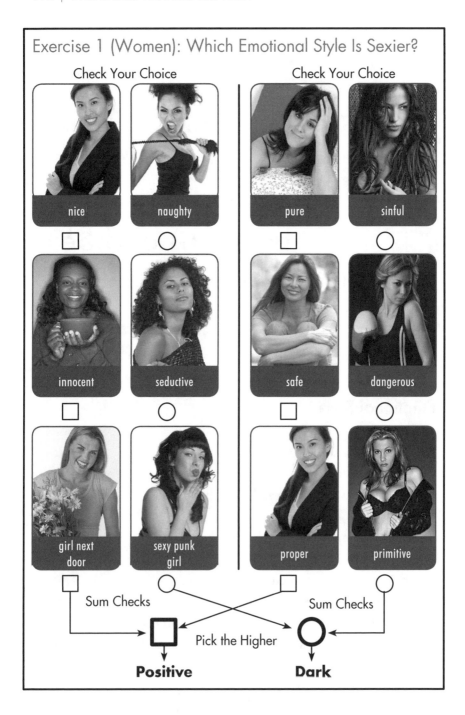

Exercise 1 (Women): Which Emotional Style Is Sexier?

Exercise 2 (Men): Which Emotional Style Is Sexier?

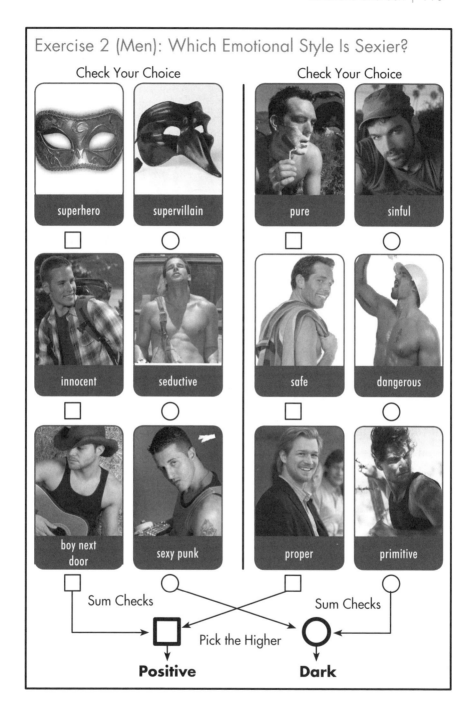

pure or sinful? safe or dangerous? Add up the number of choices you make on the left and on the right to see whether you prefer one emotional tone over another.

You may find that you're drawn to a mixture of qualities. There's nothing wrong with liking a little naughty mixed in with your nice. However, since several of the exercises in upcoming chapters ask you to pick a side, try to identify whether you are primarily drawn to positive emotions associated with sex or darker emotions.

As a tie breaker, I recommend trying the exercise that matches *your* gender and exploring how the qualities apply to you. Check the options that best describe how *you* come across in sexual situations. Are you innocent or seductive? Do you come across as proper or primitive? The sexual style you convey to other people is probably in line with the emotional part of sex you find most natural and engaging.

What Makes Darker Emotions Kinky?

As we saw in Chapter 2, the most adventurous forms of sex usually involve darker emotions. Kinky sex is especially likely to involve some element of pain, fear, or danger. Not everyone who is drawn to dark and sinful sex has Kinky tastes, however. There are plenty of folks with Mainstream tastes who are turned on by sex that is more naughty than nice. But if you meet someone with Kinky tastes, you can safely bet that he or she likes sex on the dark side and is bored and uninterested in the lighter and more wholesome side of sex.

The truth is that all sex is risky and (occasionally) painful. The threat of catching or transmitting a sexually transmitted disease hangs over the sex lives of most single men and women. Given that birth control is imperfect, even married couples have to worry about sex leading to pregnancy.

Most of us try to minimize these types of pain and risk. To most of us, the less risk and pain involved, the more comfortable we are with sex.

What sets people with Kinky tastes apart is that they intentionally seek out risk, danger, and pain. They're turned on by sex that is unpredictable. They like having sex in places where they might get caught. They like testing limits. They want sex to be messy and weird. They don't want sex to be conventional or sanitized.

What Is the Appeal of Sex Mixed with Pain?

Why would someone be drawn to sex that hurts? Why do some individuals like being whipped or paddled? Why do others enjoy having their nipples pinched or having hot wax dripped on them?

I won't pretend to understand all the motivations people have for doing what they do. However, as a clinical psychologist, I can point to three possible motivations for mixing pain with sex.

First, both pain and pleasure focus your attention. They change your priorities. When you are in pain, other worries and concerns in your mind disappear. All you can think about is what is hurting and why. Thus, pain can distract you from your work stress or other worries. Pain also focuses blood flow to the area being hurt. So a smack on the butt can really hurt, but when it's followed by a gentle kiss or caress, the soft sensation feels incredibly intense and pleasurable.

Second, our brains appear to reward the endurance of certain kinds of pain. Specifically, pain that results from physical exertion toward a goal, like the pain a ballet dancer or marathon runner endures, can lead the reward centers of the brain to release endorphins. Similarly, someone who endures pain as part of kinky sex (like being paddled) may feel a sense of pride and get a rush of endorphins, because the brain interprets the experience as a physical challenge.

Third, pain implies power. The one who delivers the pain, with a spank or a bite, is dominant over the one who receives it. As we'll see in the next chapter, the expression and experience of power as part of sex is a big turn-on to at least half of all men and women.

For these folks, pain helps reinforce who is in charge and who has to surrender.

We've now covered the first of the three components of sexual chemistry. Let's turn to the next component and the role power plays in your sexual connections.

Chapter 7

Power and Sex

What Power Dynamics Turn You On?

Expressing and Surrendering Power

What Is the Least Popular Sex Topic?

Of all the topics I cover in my sex surveys, the issue of power and sex is by far the least popular. Most men and women are hesitant to assign labels like dominant or submissive to their sexual interests. If you ask whether power plays *any* role in their enjoyment of sex, most people emphatically will say NO! and want to change the topic.

Yet when I skip the labels and simply *describe* sexual activities that involve power or control by using phrases like "taking charge" or "being on top," most people identify at least one activity that they enjoy. So before you throw up your defenses and decide that this chapter isn't relevant to you, let's look at two sets of activities that involve either the expression of power or the surrender of power during sex.

Does Expressing Power Turn You On?

Are you sexually excited when *your partner*...?

- ☐ initiates having sex
- ☐ takes charge sexually
- ☐ tells you what to do (or how to do it) sexually
- ☐ acts in an aggressive way in bed

Are you sexually excited when *you*...?

- ☐ initiate having sex
- ☐ take charge sexually
- ☐ tell your partner what to do (or how to do it) sexually
- ☐ act in an aggressive way in bed

Obviously, each of these actions is an expression of sexual control or influence. Each action is a little more forceful or dominant than the one before it.

Does Surrendering Power Turn You On?

Are you sexually excited when *your partner*...?

- ☐ surrenders to you
- ☐ serves you sexually
- ☐ is held down by you

Do you feel excited or calmed, when *you*...?

- ☐ surrender yourself to your partner
- ☐ serve your partner sexually
- ☐ are held down by your partner

What Is a Power Dynamic?

If you find *any* of these activities enjoyable, then power plays at least a small role in your enjoyment of sex. If you prefer *one* set of activities (like expressing power or surrendering power), then you have a preferred *power dynamic.* You like playing a particular role during sex, and you need a partner who can play the complementary role. It's this dynamic—the connection between what turns you on and what turns your partner on—that creates sexual chemistry in a single encounter and can be the cornerstone of long-term compatibility.

We'll look at *six* power dynamics in this chapter. Each dynamic involves a particular set of expectations for what each partner will do and will not do as part of sex. I'm going to give each dynamic a name or label (like *versatile dominant* or *versatile submissive*).

I know these labels tend to make people uncomfortable. I also don't want to oversimplify your tastes and interests by sorting you into one of the six buckets. However, we are going to need these labels in the upcoming chapters as we add more ingredients to our understanding of sexual chemistry. In Chapter 10 we'll see how power dynamics combine with other sexual interests (like enjoying lighter or darker sexual themes) to create unique sexual personas. Plus, in Chapter 11 we'll use your preferred power dynamic to find a partner who you'll click with sexually or, in Chapter 12, create a plan for improving the sexual chemistry with your current partner.

Breaking the Taboo

If understanding the connection between power and sex is so important in finding and creating good sexual chemistry, why do people feel so uncomfortable talking about it? Why is this topic taboo?

I asked hundreds of men and women this question and identified three reasons for the taboo. Let's take a look at each of the concerns. Hopefully, in the process, I can dissuade you of any misgivings you are holding onto that might prevent you from discovering your favorite sexual dynamic.

Are You Afraid Power Will Turn into Abuse?

The most common fear about power and sex is that the expression of power will somehow turn into abuse. This fear is especially common among individuals who were abused as children, who witnessed abuse between their parents, or who have been abused by a partner as an adult. Even if you've never been abused or taken advantage of, you may still have concerns about mixing sex with control or force of any kind. Since good sex often involves losing control and letting go of your inhibitions, many women (and some men) fear that things can easily get out of hand and go too far.

I believe a certain level of caution is a good thing. It is important to identify and distinguish between what constitutes *acceptable* and *unacceptable* expressions of power, and then be careful to respect these limits. For the record, violence, force, or cruelty of *any kind* should *never* be part of a relationship. You should never feel threatened or have control *taken* from you as part of sex (or in any other aspect of your relationship, for that matter). If at any point either you or your partner feels uncomfortable (even if you are unsure *why* you feel that way) you should be free to say so. Then you and your partner should either change what you are doing or take a time-out to talk about what happened.

I've interviewed couples who negotiated their limits and comfort zones without ever having to talk about them explicitly. Good for them. However, most couples need to talk about these issues explicitly. Furthermore, their comfort zones may change over time and require new conversations. Regardless, you both need to feel safe and know that the expression of power or the surrender of power will occur within the limits you both agreed to.

Are You Confused about How Men and Women Are Supposed to Relate?

In previous generations, people didn't talk about power and sex in part because gender roles (both in and out of the bedroom) were socially prescribed and usually unquestioned. Men initiated sex and played a sexually dominant role, while women played a more submissive role. Of course, by today's standards (or at least by the Kinky standards we looked at in Chapter 2), neither person played a completely dominant or submissive role. Still, there was little flexibility in terms of who could express power and who could surrender it.

After several decades of the so-called sexual revolution, traditional gender roles inside and outside of the bedroom seem passé. Today, egalitarian sex roles are assumed to be the norm. This is all good news if it frees couples to explore new roles and find a dynamic that fits the needs and desires of both partners.

However, this is not always the case. The widespread perception that sex roles are supposed to be equal has left many men and women who prefer traditional sexual roles feeling marginalized. I've interviewed numerous women *and* men who were hesitant to talk about sexual fantasies or relationships with dominant-submissive themes, because they were afraid others would judge them harshly.

I've spoken to men who have healthy, modern attitudes about gender, but they enjoy playing a dominant role sexually and worry that this implies they are sexist. I've spoken with women who are progressive and modern in every way, but they enjoy playing a submissive role sexually and worry that this means they are maladjusted.

So if you're confused about gender roles and unsure about how men and women are supposed to relate, you are not alone. The struggle for gender equality is about the freedom to choose. As a couple, it means the freedom to decide as individuals how you want to relate sexually, without having to follow a predetermined script.

The Appeal of an Older Man

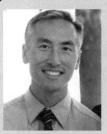

About one in five young women say they are attracted to middle-aged or older men. Although they may date men their own age, many say they would choose a more confident and experienced man any night of the week. A mature man has a lot to offer:

1. **Power.** You don't have to own an oil company to be powerful. Power is about being comfortable with yourself and confident about what you have to offer. A powerful man doesn't have to prove himself or brag about what he has or who he knows. His accomplishments speak for themselves. Power means not being afraid of rejection. He understands that being turned down says nothing about his value as a person. That kind of cool confidence is very sexy.

2. **Substance.** Younger women talk a lot about the importance of authenticity. Most women are impressed by a man who knows who he is and what he believes. A mature man doesn't play games or try to be someone he is not in order to impress women.

    Younger guys spend a lot of time on dates talking about what they are going to do...someday. As one young woman put it: "Boys who are still trying to figure out what they want to be when they grow up are boring." A mature man has already built a life and has something to show for his efforts.

3. **Skills.** Yes, it's true. A woman likes a man with skills. She doesn't want to waste a night with a man who can't find her clitoris or who thinks foreplay consists of taking his pants off. A mature man knows what he's doing in bed and enjoys pleasing women. Frankly, young men are often a little afraid of vaginas. A woman would rather be with a man who loves and appreciates her body.

Do You Assume Power Is Masculine?

The other piece of cultural baggage we bring with us from the last century is a perception that equates power with masculinity. In study after study, I've found that most women view men who are powerful because of their status, wealth, or prestige as more attractive than men with less power. This is one of the reasons why one in five young women (under the age of twenty-five) find successful middle-aged or older men sexy. See, for example, the sidebar "The Appeal of an Older Man."

The problem this creates for both men and women is that power is often *only* associated with masculinity. Power is not seen as a feminine quality. In study after study, I've found that most men do *not* view women who are powerful because of their status, wealth, or prestige as more attractive or sexy than women with less power. In fact, almost half the men in my studies said that power actually made a woman *less* appealing in their eyes.

To illustrate how this prejudice gets in the way, let me tell you about the romance between Tom and Tracey. When I give lectures on this topic, I always draw a brick wall in the middle of the blackboard, and I name the wall "Power Is Masculine." On one side of the wall I write "feminine" and on the other I write "masculine," because this prejudice acts like a wall that divides the sexual world into these two domains. Next, I draw a female stick figure (named Tracey) on the feminine side of the blackboard. Then I draw a male stick figure (named Tom) on the masculine side of the board. Both Tracey and Tom were raised to believe that power is masculine, and they accept the wall between them.

Tom and Tracey start to date, and a romance blossoms. Tom asks her out on a Friday night, and Tracey thinks this is the night they will finally go all the way. However, Tom is extremely shy, so Tracey decides she is going to have to make the first move sexually.

When Tracey thinks about how she is going to initiate sex, she realizes that this is an action on the masculine side of the wall. That night, when she tries to initiate sex, it feels unnatural. A voice inside her head tells her that this is not the sort of thing a proper and respectable lady does. So, unfortunately, Tom and Tracey's romantic evening goes nowhere.

The next night, Tracey decides she has to tear down the wall, let go of her old-fashioned hang-ups, and get naked with shy Tom. Unfortunately, Tom still has his "power is masculine" beliefs and sees Tracey's actions as *taking* an activity from his masculine domain. He feels emasculated, robbed of power, and impotent. So nothing happens on Saturday night either.

Obviously, this is an exaggerated scenario. I'm describing these thoughts and actions as if they were conscious decisions. However, in most situations, prejudices are implicit and operate outside of our conscious awareness. Still, this basic scenario captures a lot of the inhibitions and anxieties that couples experience when women act sexually assertive and men try to surrender control to their partner. I can tell you from my clinical experience of doing couple's therapy and sex therapy that many men who struggle with erectile dysfunction attribute the problem to feeling emasculated in the bedroom, in their relationship, or both.

Let's give up on Tom and Tracey and meet two other couples. Let's add a male stick figure on the masculine side of the board and call him Eddie. Eddie enjoys letting go sexually and surrendering to women. However, since Eddie was taught that power is masculine, he's afraid that surrendering power will make him feminine. So he's afraid to show this side of himself to his wife. Instead, Eddie enjoys monthly visits to a prostitute named Clarissa.

At this point, I draw a dominatrix stick figure of Clarissa on the feminine side of the board. Eddie has learned that he can let himself go sexually and surrender sexually *if* he is forced to do so as part of role-play. He doesn't feel comfortable going on the other side of the wall voluntarily. However, if Clarissa ties him up and drags him over the wall, he can surrender without losing his masculinity. In other words, he can only lose control when it is *taken* from him.

Again, this is an extreme example. Still, as you'll see in Chapters 9 and 12, themes of surrendering power through force pop up again and again in heterosexual men's fantasies and their favorite role-play scenarios. An interesting study of requests made to prostitutes and call girls found that dominatrix role-play is especially popular among conservative men with high-pressure jobs. These men only feel comfortable losing control to a dark and powerful woman who uses confinement and punishment to force him into submission.[25]

Let's draw one final couple on the board. On the feminine side, let's add a female stick figure and call her Sharon. She's in her early forties, she's fit, and she has a great career. Sharon has a twenty-something admirer named Josh.

The popular press has labeled older women like Sharon who date younger men as "cougars." This implies a predatory power dynamic. However, I've found in my studies that most May-December romances involve younger men who pursue older woman, and not the other way around (see the sidebar "The Appeal of an Older Woman").

Let's assume that Sharon is resistant at first to Josh's advances, but eventually she gives in and they start a romance. The two develop a mentor-pupil dynamic sexually. Josh defers to Sharon, who takes the lead sexually and shares her sexual wisdom.

How is it that Josh feels comfortable with a more powerful female partner? Perhaps Josh doesn't believe in the "power is masculine" stereotype. Another possible explanation is that Josh entered the relationship already accepting and admiring Sharon's personal power. Since Sharon is already powerful in his mind, she is not taking away from his masculinity when she takes the lead sexually.

The Appeal of an Older Woman

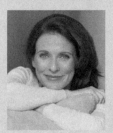

Love affairs between young men and middle-aged or older women are in vogue. Sharon Stone and Demi Moore have paved the way for other May-December romances and for good reason. If you're a woman of a certain age who's attracted to a younger man but need some extra motivation, keep the following three things in mind:

1. **Her skills.** A mature woman's sexual skills are a big turn-on for younger guys. She has more experience with men than the girls he is used to. She will know how to push his buttons in ways he has never experienced.

   She also brings a lot of experience with her own body. She knows what she enjoys and can show him how to please a woman fully. He will like that she knows what she's doing. Most young men are eager to become pupils to a more mature teacher.

2. **Take charge.** Younger men are typically more open than middle-aged or older men to having a woman take charge sexually. Young men get tired of always being the one who has to make the first move. Most young guys will be flattered by your advances and gladly be seduced.

   Remember, confidence is sexy. Younger guys often complain that women expect them to read their minds and magically know how to please them. If you're the more mature partner, take a firm hand and show him how to release your magic.

3. **Uninhibited.** Young men are eager to please. They get bored with women their own age who are often uncomfortable with their bodies and unfamiliar with the wilder and more exciting aspects of sex. Younger guys enjoy a woman who is less inhibited and more responsive. So don't be afraid to moan or be vocal with your pleasure. Seeing and hearing you in ecstasy will be a big turn-on to your future boy toy.

Can You Let Go of These Prejudices and Taboos?

To sum up, a number of societal shifts have left many people feeling confused about the connection between sex and power. My point of view is that any combination of power (including dominance or submission) is acceptable as long as *both* adults agree to the activities and respect and protect each other's limits and safety.[26]

If you're single, the challenge is to find a partner who wants the same power dynamic that you want. The good news is that, no matter what you enjoy, there are plenty of others out there who enjoy it as well. You simply have to understand what you want, what your partner wants, and be able to talk about it.

If you're in a relationship, you have to assess the power dynamics that each of you prefers and then see how well they fit (or clash). As long as there is some versatility in your tastes, there are ways to accommodate both of your sexual interests. You may not be able to satisfy both of your needs at the same time, but you can find a way to take turns and be satisfied with your sex life as a whole.

To help you get there, let's turn to two sets of exercises. We start at the surface level, with exercises that focus on the external qualities that relate to power. We'll see whether you're drawn to powerful or gentle personas. Then, we'll look at your favorite sexual activities and explore whether you are turned on by dominant or submissive sexual roles.

Power Dynamics

Are You Powerful or Gentle?

One of the core messages you broadcast to the world each day has to do with your personal power. The way you look, dress, walk, and talk tells a story about how powerful (potent, strong, dominant, influential) or weak (fragile, vulnerable, submissive) you see yourself.

Western societies tend to assume:

Power = Good

Weakness = Bad

Yet, not every society makes these same assumptions. Power is expressed and interpreted differently in other cultures. In most Asian cultures, for example, a bold and assertive person is typically viewed as a braggart and assumed to be weak, while a quiet and reserved person is assumed to be strong. The power dimensions discussed in this chapter are largely independent from the emotional dimensions of sex we covered in the last chapter. Not all powerful traits are positive or good and not all weak traits are negative or bad.

In fact, a number of *weak* traits have *positive* connotations and are usually seen as appealing or attractive. They include being innocent, dutiful, respectful, modest, youthful, and virginal.

Powerful attributes with *positive* connotations also tend to have universal appeal. They include being confident, competitive, courageous, competent, and charming. These traits are usually at the top of the wish list for what most men and many women are looking for in an ideal partner.

So try to approach Exercises 1 and 2 with an open mind. Let's start by exploring how you see yourself. Look at the exercise that matches your gender. There are six pairs of descriptions. Put a check under the quality that best describes you. Then total the checks you made in the squares and the checks you made in the circles. If you identify with the choices on the left (the squares), you probably have a *powerful* personal presence. If you identify with the options on the right (the circles), you probably have a *gentle* personal style.

If you're a man and you identify with the *powerful* qualities, then you have a gender-typical profile. Similarly, if you're a woman and you identify with the *gentle* qualities, then you have a gender-typical profile. Being gender-typical simply means you're aligned with

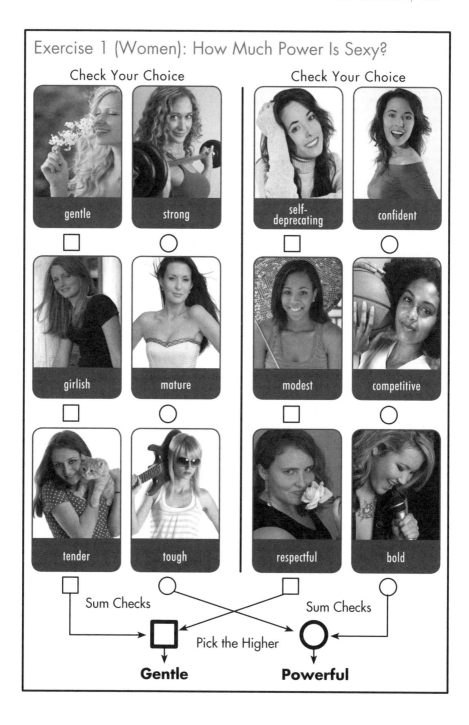

Exercise 1 (Women): How Much Power Is Sexy?

Check Your Choice　　　　Check Your Choice

gentle　strong　self-deprecating　confident

girlish　mature　modest　competitive

tender　tough　respectful　bold

Sum Checks　　Sum Checks

Pick the Higher

Gentle　**Powerful**

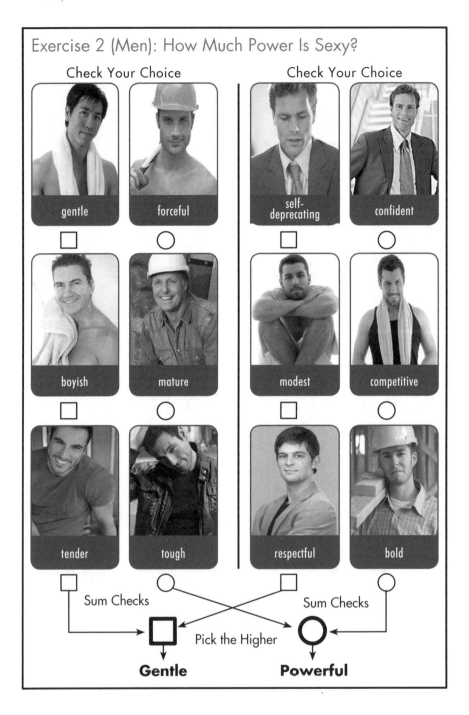

Exercise 2 (Men): How Much Power Is Sexy?

Check Your Choice · Check Your Choice

gentle · forceful · self-deprecating · confident

boyish · mature · modest · competitive

tender · tough · respectful · bold

Sum Checks · Sum Checks

Pick the Higher

Gentle · **Powerful**

what society tends to expect of men and women. To take this a step further, ask yourself for each option: what is a man or woman *supposed* to be? There are no right or wrong answers. However, the more you associate power with masculinity and gentleness with femininity, the more "locked in" you may be to your power dynamic.

Are You Drawn to Powerful or Gentle Lovers?

Now take a look at the exercise that matches the gender you're attracted to. Ask yourself for each pair of descriptions: which quality do you find sexier? If you consistently favor the right option in each of the six pairs, you are probably drawn to a strong or powerful personal style. If you favor the options on the left, you probably prefer a weaker or gentler style.

These are all *external* qualities, but your preferences here tend to offer a window into your sexual interests. If you have a strong preference for one set of options over another, then the chances are very good that we will see these preferences pop up again in your sexual power dynamics.

Which Sexual Power Dynamic Do You Prefer?

Now that we've explored your general attitude toward power and attraction, let's look at what you actually like to do sexually. At the start of the chapter, I asked whether you enjoyed taking charge sexually, surrendering sexually, doing both, or doing neither. Now let's look at these options again and see how different sexual interests combine to create six power dynamics.

Take a moment to complete either Exercise 3 (for women) or Exercise 4 (for men). The exercises ask who you want to initiate sex and branch through two sets of options regarding your role and your partner's role during sex. The charts end with six power dynamics. If we collapse the three versatile categories (versatile,

Exercise 3: Power Dynamics for Women

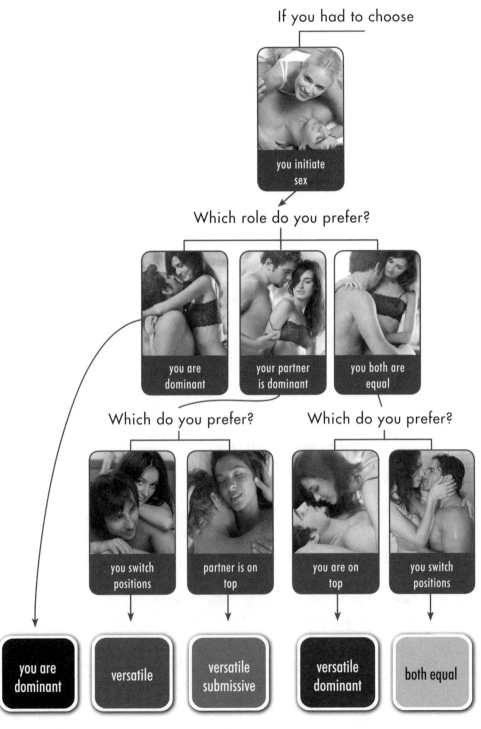

which would you prefer?

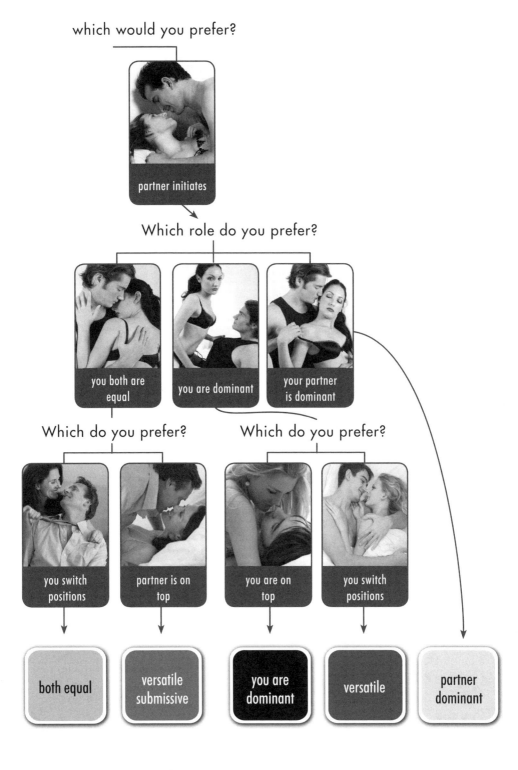

Exercise 4: Power Dynamics for Men

If you had to choose

you initiate
sex

Which role do you prefer?

you are
dominant

your partner
is dominant

you both are
equal

Which do you prefer?

Which do you prefer?

you switch
positions

partner is on
top

you are on
top

you switch
positions

you are
dominant

versatile

versatile
submissive

versatile
dominant

both equal

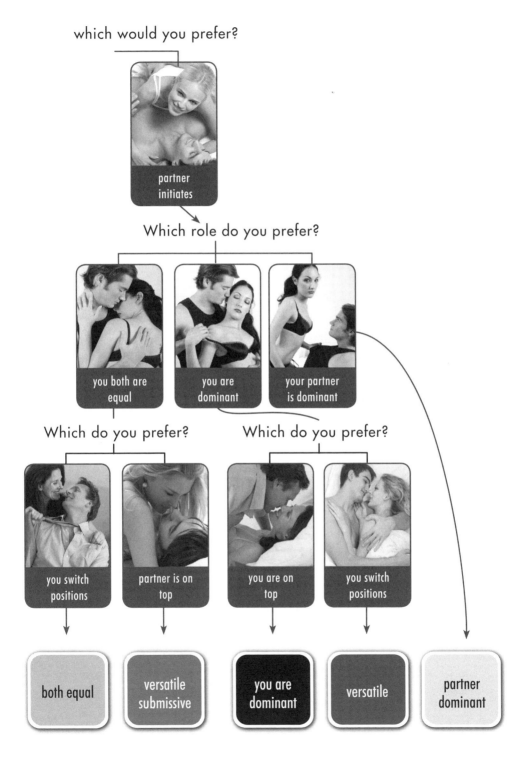

versatile-submissive, and versatile-dominant) into a single category, it leaves us with four main dynamics.

The following is a description of the power dynamics and the most compatible partner for each. Also, take a look at the pie charts in Figure 1 and the proportion of men and women who fit in each of the power dynamics.[27] See how common (or rare) your own preferred dynamic is compared to other men and women.

You Are Dominant (Partner Is Submissive)

You prefer to take the lead sexually. You like to take charge of *what* you do and *when* you do it. You set the pace for sex and enjoy bringing your partner to orgasm. Some dominant lovers express their power by being very verbal and directing the sexual action. Others take charge through their body language and movement. Obviously, the most compatible lover for you is a more submissive partner who enjoys and appreciates your skills and desires.

About one in twenty women (6 percent) and one in ten men (12 percent) are sexually dominant. Thus, although this is an extreme preference and is not highly popular overall, it is twice as common among men as it is women.

Now let's look at the opposite end of the spectrum.

Partner Is Dominant (You Are Submissive)

You enjoy having a partner who takes the lead sexually. You enjoy being able to let go and let your partner guide the experience.

Figure 1: Breakdown of Power Dynamics for Women and Men

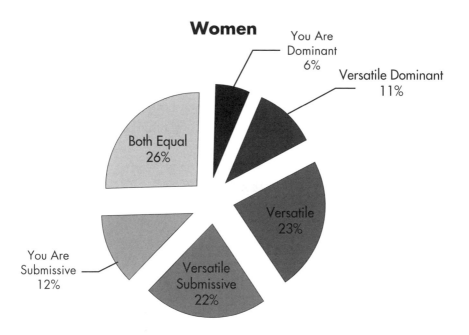

Women

You Are Dominant 6%

Versatile Dominant 11%

Versatile 23%

Versatile Submissive 22%

You Are Submissive 12%

Both Equal 26%

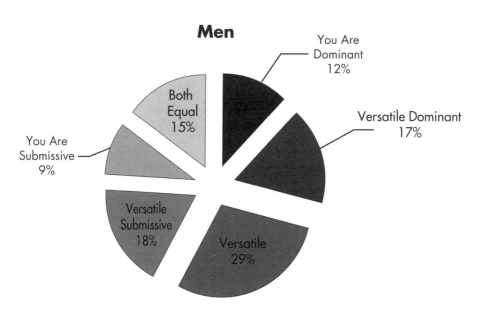

Men

You Are Dominant 12%

Versatile Dominant 17%

Versatile 29%

Versatile Submissive 18%

You Are Submissive 9%

Both Equal 15%

Like most men and women who prefer more dominant partners, you are probably a generous and giving lover. You enjoy pleasing your partner. It's exciting when your partner tells you what to do or directs you with his or her hands.

About one in ten women (12 percent) and men (9 percent) prefer their partner to be dominant. So this extreme preference is somewhat rare, but it is equally common among both men and women.

Next, we look at individuals who fall in the middle of the sexual power spectrum.

Versatile Dominant or Submissive

You enjoy changing roles between encounters or within the same encounter. You are skilled at both taking and surrendering sexual control. Depending on the strength of your preferences, you may be versatile but lean toward expressing or surrendering power.

A *versatile-dominant* person can switch roles but leans toward being dominant. Slightly more men are versatile-dominant (17 percent) than women (11 percent).

Similarly, a *versatile-submissive* person is also flexible but leans toward a more submissive dynamic. About one in five women (22 percent) and men (18 percent) fit this description.

Finally, there are purely versatile individuals who equally enjoy playing dominant and submissive roles. About one in five women (22 percent) and one in three men (29 percent) fit this description.

Taken together, the vast majority of men and women fall in one of these midrange preference categories.

To complicate matters, your style of versatility can be expressed in different ways. Versatility can either be expressed by switching roles on different occasions or by switching roles within an encounter.

If you fit the first approach, you enjoy playing a dominant role in one encounter, but then you want to switch roles and play a submissive role the next time. For you, it's probably easier to stay in a single role, rather than have to shift gears or change your mind-set during the same encounter. If you take charge, you like to be in complete control. If you surrender, you want to let go completely. The ideal partner for you has the same style of versatility. Being with someone who is entirely dominant or entirely submissive will fit only some, but not all, of your desires.

Alternatively, you may enjoy being versatile *within* the same encounter. If so, you enjoy a lot of give and take with your partner. To you, the expression of power during sex is a fluid process. You have no problem shifting gears. For you, a compatible lover would share your ability to switch roles spontaneously.

Finally, we turn to individuals who do not fit any of the above power dynamics.

Both Equal

You have a very egalitarian approach to sex and tend to prefer sex *without* a strong expression of power from either partner. Being with a dominant partner (or having a partner who expects *you* to play a dominant role) probably makes you feel uncomfortable. For you, sex is a sensual experience. You do not look to sex as a means to release stress or express emotional intensity.

Your ideal lover would share this approach to sex and not need you to play either a dominant or submissive role in order to be sexually satisfied.

About one in four women (26 percent) and one in seven men (15 percent) fit this egalitarian approach to sex.

Do You and Your Partner Have Compatible Power Dynamics?

If you're in a relationship, I recommend you complete Exercises 3 and 4 from a few different points of view. First, choose the options that reflect your *current* sexual dynamic with your partner: what roles do you and your partner currently play? Second, complete the exercise while thinking of your *ideal* sexual connection: what role would you play in an ideal sexual relationship? Finally, complete the exercise by thinking of how your partner might answer if he or she were totally honest about what turns him or her on: what role would your partner play in an ideal sexual relationship?

Obviously, the more aligned these three outcomes are, the more compatible your relationship is. The more your *current* dynamic differs from *your* ideal or *your partner's* ideal, the bigger the challenge you face in creating a compatible relationship. As we'll see in Chapter 12, there are ways of addressing even dramatic mismatches. But for now, don't worry about fixing any inconsistencies; just *describe* the situation. We still have a few more steps before we can paint a complete picture of your strengths and challenges.

What Are Some of the Myths about Sex and Power?

Sexual dynamics can obviously be pretty complicated. It is important not to confuse power dynamics with preferences for specific sexual *activities.* A lot of the myths about power and sex center on false ideas we have about how dominant and submissive lovers are supposed to behave. Here are a few of the most common misperceptions.

MYTH: All dominant men are obsessed with intercourse, have to be on top, prefer sex to be rough and fast, and are not concerned with their partner's orgasm.

FACT: Men with dominant or versatile-dominant sexual styles like the same range of activities as men with other preferred dynamics. Men who prefer a dominant role are often very giving lovers, enjoy oral sex, and can prefer slow and tender sex.

There are two common misconceptions about women and power.

MYTH: All dominant women enjoy playing a dominatrix.

FACT: Only dominant women with Kinky sexual tastes (see Chapter 2) would fit what most of us think of as a dominatrix. A dominant woman with Vanilla sexual tastes may simply enjoy being on top of her lover during intercourse or enjoy guiding her lover during sex.

MYTH: All submissive women are passive and sexually boring.

FACT: Submissive women can be very passionate and active lovers and simply prefer to have a partner who initiates and guides their sexual activity.

How Do Emotions and Power Combine?

In Chapter 6 we looked at the emotional tone of sex. We explored whether you prefer sex with a light emotional tone (that is, positive, wholesome, and joyful) or sex with a dark emotional tone (that is, sinful, naughty, or dirty). Now that we've described sexual power dynamics, we've covered two of the three ingredients to sexual chemistry. In Chapters 9 and 10, we'll see how all three facets of sexual chemistry combine to create unique sexual fantasy zones and personas.

As a preview, let's see how emotional tone and the two extreme power dynamics combine to create different types of lovers with very different sexual interests. Take a look at Exercise 5. Pick one of the two emotional styles and the power dynamic that is closest to your tastes. Then see if the description of that combination fits your style. If so, then we're on the right track. If not, and you prefer a *versatile* dynamic, don't worry. We'll get to your unique tastes in the next several chapters.

Once you've found the description that is closest to your style, look at the style directly above or directly below yours. This type of lover would probably be a compatible match. If you're more submissive, you obviously need a more dominant partner, and vice versa. If you and your partner both want to play the same role or prefer different emotional tones, your sexual styles are going to clash. As we'll see in Chapter 12, this doesn't have to be a deal breaker, but it's important to know where your challenges are coming from so you can talk about them honestly and openly.

What Is the Most Challenging Clash to Deal With?

If you prefer sex with a lighter emotional tone and do *not* enjoy playing dominant or submissive roles to the extreme, then the good news is that you're like the majority of men and women. The chances are favorable that most of the potential partners you will meet will fall into a similar sexual zone. The biggest challenge you face is ending up with a partner who is turned on by more extreme power dynamics with darker emotional tones.

Why do these men and women seem so weird? They've found ways to eroticize certain taboo roles and behaviors that the rest of us try to avoid. Most of us spend our lives trying to avoid being humiliated, for example. Yet people with Kinky tastes who are also submissive often enjoy being symbolically humiliated and even literally spat upon. Being insulted and criticized as part of role-play strips away one's ego and pretenses. A man or woman with a high pressure job, for example, may find being told "you're a worthless dog" helps him or her forget about work responsibilities, frees inhibitions, and lets him or her live fully in the moment. If so, good for you!

Similarly, few of us would ever consider fear to be an attractive quality in a partner. However, it's not uncommon for people to

Exercise 5: Combining Power and Emotion

	Do You Enjoy the Lighter or Darker Side of Sex?	
Which Role Do You Prefer to Play?	**Lighter Tone**	**Darker Tone**
More Submissive	**Submissive Light** **Lovers are...** *Attentive, dutiful,* and *innocent.* They enjoy playing the *novice, pupil,* or *sexual servant.*	**Submissive Dark** **Lovers are...** *Obedient, naughty,* and *mischievous.* They enjoy role-play where they are *forced* to serve their partner. Some like to *struggle* or feign *protest* to heighten the intensity of the experience.
More Dominant	**Dominant Light** **Lovers are...** *Playful, fun,* and *exciting.* They enjoy *guiding, directing,* and *protecting* their lover.	**Dominant Dark** **Lovers are...** *Strong, strict, rough,* and *forceful.* They enjoy giving *orders* and *commands* and role-play where they can *punish* and *discipline* their partner.

take dates to horror movies, knowing that he or she may grab your shoulder (or maybe even jump in your lap) during the scary scenes. Similarly, dark emotional role-play (with leather and maybe even a play dungeon) creates fear in one partner and puts the dominant partner in the role of protector or savior.

Then there are sex slaves. Wars have been fought so that no man or woman would ever have to be a slave. Yet a number of Kinky men and women not only want to be submissive, they want to become their partner's slave. In addition to borrowing the term *slave*, the Kinky subculture has also eroticized many slavery icons, including chains, collars, and whips. At the furthest extreme, some couples even role-play selling or swapping their slave partner with other couples.

The moral of this story, boys and girls, is that the same core power dynamic can be expressed in myriad ways depending upon one's favorite sexual activities and your preferred emotional tone. The story has already started to get complicated, and we haven't even considered the interplay between power dynamics and the intensity of sex. Let's turn to this third ingredient of sexual chemistry and explore the intensity, speed, and flow of sex that you enjoy.

Chapter 8

Sex and Intensity

Do You Like It Fast or Slow?

Your Sexual Journey

Do You Prefer a Fast Journey or a Slow Journey?

You've probably heard the saying, "It's not the size of the boat; it's the motion of the ocean." Whether or not you agree with this penis-size metaphor, I think we can all agree that motion definitely matters. Each person's idea about what constitutes great versus mediocre sex usually refers to a specific level of activity and style of movement.

Most sexual fantasies and sexual encounters end at a similar place: an exciting climax. But the sexual journey, or *how* you get there, differs. For the sake of illustration, let's call one a *fast* journey and the other a *slow* journey.

The *fast* journey is about intensity, excitement, change, and movement. Sex involves a lot of different sexual activities. Clothes are stripped off and thrown around the room. Kissing is deep and passionate. There's a lot of rolling around, flipping between sexual positions, and maybe even switching rooms a few times. Excitement and arousal start high and stay high throughout. It's a hot and sweaty good time.

The *slow* journey is leisurely, sensual, relaxing, and focused. If the fast journey is about quantity, the slow journey is about quality. There is a gradual progression, where each activity is enjoyed and savored. Touching is gentle. Kisses are soft. There is no agenda, required destination, or timetable. Each lover is very focused on the other. Both feel comfortable, relaxed, and free from pressure.

These descriptions represent anchors on a slow to fast sexual activity continuum. You may enjoy switching between styles on different occasions or even mixing styles within an encounter. Nevertheless, chances are you probably gravitate toward one style or the other. When people describe their ideal lovers and sexual fantasies, they also tend to describe a single place along the activity continuum.

If it's difficult for you to describe your sexual style or the style you find attractive in broad terms, think about how you approach particular kinds of sexual activity, like foreplay. What style of touch do you find most arousing? Some people are turned on by a soft and slow touch; the slower and more sensual the better. Others like to be held and touched in a fast, deep, and intense way. Does your style of touching or kissing reflect your broader approach to sex?

Which Activity Style Are You Drawn To?

To help you determine which activity style you find most appealing, Exercises 1 and 2 present multiple pairs of fast and slow activity descriptions. First, complete the exercise with photos of your preferred gender. Pick the type of connection you find most appealing. If you had to pick, would you rather have a partner who is relaxing or exciting to be with? Are you more drawn to a partner who is affectionate or energetic? You can look at these as general traits or as qualities specific to the type of sex you enjoy. Either way, I believe your choices will point to the type of sexual style you find most attractive.

You can also complete the exercise with the photos that match your own gender and pick the options that best describe your own energy. If you had to pick, would you say your style is more comfortable or playful? Are you focused sexually or do you like to change and switch around your attention sexually? Hopefully, you'll see a pattern that describes your personal sexual style.

Most of the time, men and women tend to be attracted to partners with similar sexual styles. If you bring a fast intensity to sex, you probably want a partner who is playful and active as well. However, there are times when opposites attract. Occasionally, people with slow and leisurely styles, for example, will be attracted to partners who are more energetic and exciting. There's no right style or wrong style. There's no right way to match styles either. For now, simply recognize what you like and what you're looking for. We'll get to the pragmatics of finding (or creating) compatible sexual styles in Part 4.

Are Men Faster Sexually and Women Slower?

Our ideas about gender and what men and women are supposed to be like tend to influence our expectations about sexual activity styles. Cultural stereotypes tend to associate *men* with *high* activity and *women* with *low* activity. These are deeply entrenched biases.

Art historian John Berger, for example, saw this at work in his study of nude paintings in Western art. He found that male nudes were usually defined by action—what he can do to you or for you.[28] Female nudes, in contrast, were typically portrayed as passive objects being observed. A number of feminist scholars have made similar observations about pornography, pointing out that women are usually portrayed as passive rather than active, as objects rather than actors.

Exercise 1 (Women): Which Activity Style Is Sexier?

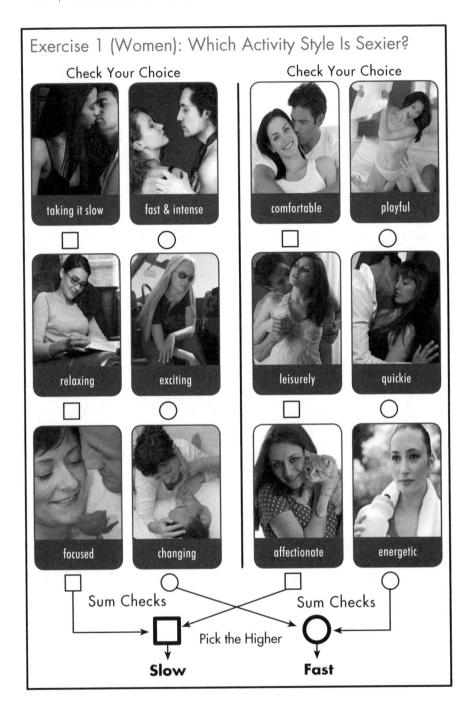

Exercise 2 (Men): Which Activity Style Is Sexier?

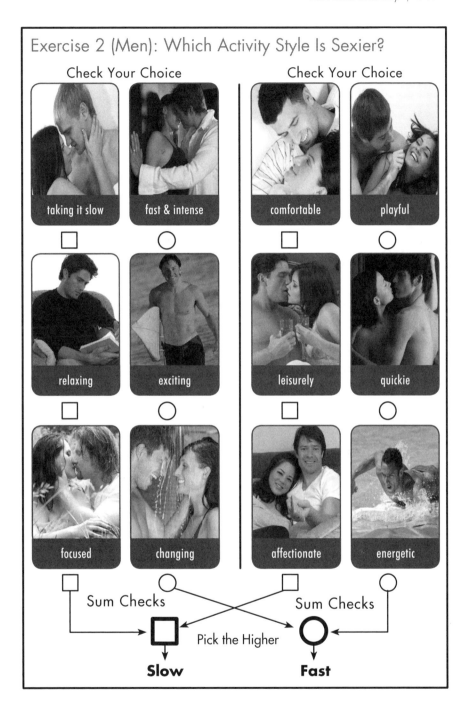

Check Your Choice   Check Your Choice

taking it slow   fast & intense   comfortable   playful

relaxing   exciting   leisurely   quickie

focused   changing   affectionate   energetic

Sum Checks   Sum Checks

Pick the Higher

Slow   **Fast**

In real life, there are men and women at both ends of the activity continuum and at all points in between. Still, in my research, I have noted a modest trend where there are slightly more men with active sexual styles and slightly more women with slower styles.

Some have pointed to physiological differences, suggesting that women may lean toward a slower style because they take longer than men to become fully aroused. However, I believe this confuses the *timing* of arousal with *what* is arousing.

No doubt, most men tend to be faster out of the gate. Women usually take a little longer to become fully aroused, to lubricate, and to orgasm. Yet what sparks arousal and what keeps it going are separate issues. Some women are more likely to be aroused by fast and intense play, while others are more likely to be aroused by slow and tender play. Similarly, many men are initially aroused by fast play, but there's also a large segment of men who are overwhelmed by too much sensation, too soon, and are more aroused by soft kissing and gentle strokes.

Your Overall Arousability

How Arousable Are You?

I believe our sexual styles are connected to our general sensitivity to stimulation or our overall *arousability*. Your sensitivity to touch, sights, sounds, and smells helps shape how much arousal you like and how you interpret different kinds of arousal. Differences in arousability can help explain why some couples are turned on by having sex outside, while others prefer to keep sex in their darkened bedroom. It can help explain why quickies are fun for some couples but a high-pressure disaster for others.

In order to understand how your body deals with arousal, it's important to know that our minds and our bodies experience emotions in very different ways. Our minds are good at distinguishing and labeling different emotions. We consciously know the difference between being excited, lustful, or afraid. However, it turns out that our bodies do not have unique physiological reactions to each of these emotional states.

So, what goes on in your body when you are surprised, turned on, or frightened can be very similar. In each case, your heart rate is elevated, your pupils dilate, all your senses are heightened, and so forth.

Let's call this underlying bodily state "arousal." It turns out that some individuals are more easily aroused than others. Their bodies remain at a more heightened state of readiness to react. For example, I typically jump a foot in the air every time the phone rings. But I have friends who are seemingly immune to almost any surprise, excitement, or threat.

To explore your arousability, take a moment to complete Exercise 3. Use the 1 to 9 scale to record how viewing each of the images makes you feel. It probably seems strange to think that seeing a river can make you feel one way or another. However, much of our mind and body operates in a realm outside of words and language. Seeing an object like a stack of money brings to mind a whole network of images, emotions, and memories. You may also notice how the thought of certain scenes or situations (like a walk in the woods) can relax you, while others (like rock climbing) can excite you.

I picked these particular images because they've proven in research to be good indicators of your sensitivity to sensations and your overall arousability.[29] Go ahead and do the exercise now. Then, total your ratings. (Don't read ahead. That's cheating!)

The rocky stream is the most calming image, and the swimmer with the shark is the most arousing. Looking at your ratings as a whole, you can use the exercise key to see whether the sum of your ratings falls into the average arousal range or whether your reaction is lower or higher than average.

Another way to approach this exercise is simply to ask yourself

Exercise 3: How Arousable Are You?

How does each image make you feel? Place your 1 to 9 ratings in the circles. Then, sum your ratings.

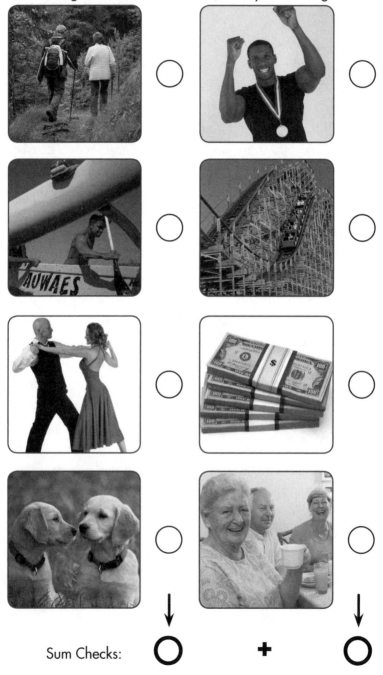

Sum Checks: ◯ **+** ◯

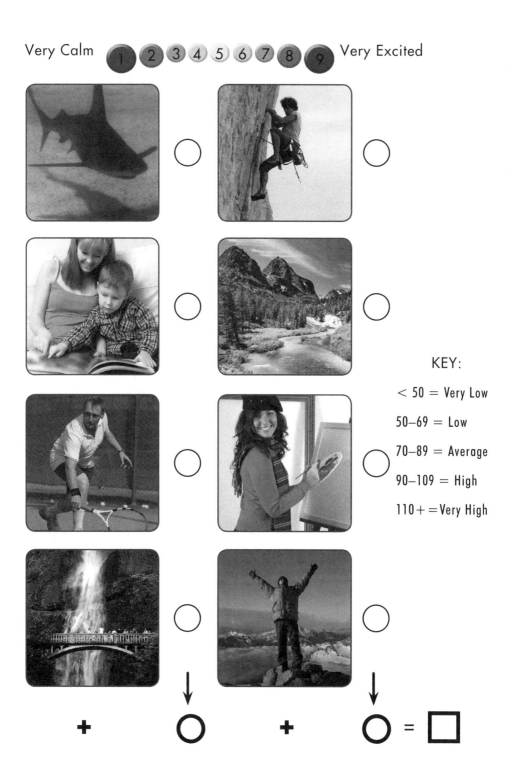

how you've reacted to being in similar situations (walks in nature, riding roller coasters, dancing, and so forth). How did your reactions to these situations compare with the reactions of your friends or family? Are you more or less prone to excitement than others?

Hopefully, between the exercise and considering your own personal experience, you have some insight into your overall level of arousal. Next, let's consider how *low* levels of arousal and *high* levels of arousal can impact people's sexual styles and their interest in particular sexual activities, like Kinky sex.

How Does Low Arousability Affect Your Sex Life?

If you are unflappable, if nothing much rattles you, then your overall arousal level may be lower than average. If this low reactivity carries over into your sex life, it can be expressed in a couple of different ways. Compared to other people, you may simply need more sexual stimulation to get excited. If this is the case, you may seek out fast and intense sexual stimulations in order to activate all your senses and fully immerse yourself in sex.

Some individuals with low arousability also seek out scenarios that most people would find scary or dangerous. Take another look at the images in Exercise 3. You'll notice that some of the images, like the photos of the roller coaster and the shark, provoke both positive and negative feelings. As you know, it's possible for something to be both exciting and scary or both beautiful and dangerous.

People with low arousability are often drawn to darker and faster sexual styles. If you enjoy scary movies, you already know that sometimes it's fun to be frightened. Having a strong dark emotional response like this can be enjoyable. If you enjoy skateboarding, rock climbing, or other adventure sports, you also know that danger can be exhilarating. Excitement is a great antidote to boredom.

People with low arousal reactions find it easier to tolerate intense arousal and tend to appreciate a mixture of positive and negative emotions. In other words, they can enjoy pleasurable sensations without being pushed away by negative ones. Similarly, people with low arousability often seek out S&M (sadism and masochism), BDSM (bondage and discipline, sadism and masochism), sex in public places, or other Kinky activities because they provoke a higher total level of arousal and because they find it easier to distinguish the pleasurable sensations from the unpleasant ones.

How Does High Arousability Affect Your Sex Life?

If you are on the other end of the arousal continuum and are easily excited, surprised, or frightened, you may be especially sensitive to the world around you and react more quickly and more intensely than most people. Negative sensations may drown out more positive ones. So, for example, looking at a photo of a shark may provoke more feelings of fear and dread than interest and excitement.

Highly sensitive people tend to like sex in settings where they can focus their attention on their lover and not have too many distractions. They usually shy away from more adventurous sex, especially if it involves pain or fear.

There are certain exceptions to this trend. In some cases, highly sensitive men and women are still drawn to adventurous experiences, despite their anxiety. A guy like this may really want to go skydiving and force himself to see it through, despite being scared to death the entire time. A woman like this may want to experiment with Kinky sex, then change her mind because the experience is too intense, but then change her mind again and want to try it. Such individuals are often caught in the push and pull between their sexual interests and their heightened sensitivity.

Again, there is nothing wrong with having mixed feelings or wanting two seemingly incompatible things. Knowing what you want and why you want it is the first step toward getting it.

Chapter 9

Sexual Fantasies

What Do Yours Reveal?

Your Sexual Fantasy Landscape

What Are Your Two Sex Lives?

Each of us has two sex lives. For most of this book we've primarily focused on your external sex life—the sexual fun you have with your partner (or partners). But we each also have an inner sex life that includes our sexual thoughts and fantasies and the time we spend masturbating.

In this chapter, we'll explore the landscape of your inner sex life. We'll see how the three facets of sexual chemistry (emotion, power, and activity) combine to create eight sexual zones. I've asked thousands of men and women to describe their favorite sexual fantasies and to place their fantasy partners, settings, and activities into these zones.

We'll identify where your fantasies fit in this sexual landscape. Then I'll present a framework for explaining why certain fantasies appeal to particular individuals and how our minds find creative ways to arouse us despite our fears and insecurities about sex.

Your fantasies offer a window into your deepest sexual desires and fears. They show us what you want sex to be and the obstacles you see standing in your way.

What Is Your Core or Primary Sexual Fantasy?

In Chapter 5, I asked you to describe your ideal lover, your ideal setting for sex, and your favorite sexual activities and roles using three rating bars for emotional tone, power, and activity. Now that we've looked at each of these dimensions separately, I suggest you go back and do that exercise again. Think about your ideal *fantasy* lover, fantasy setting, and fantasy sexual roles.

Most people have a core or primary sexual fantasy that they've enjoyed for years. It's like a reliable friend whom you can always count on to deliver. Fantasies about particular people or situations may come and go, but your *primary* fantasy involves a particular scenario that (for whatever reason) always excites you.

When individuals have had a difficult time identifying a favorite fantasy, I have described it like this: Imagine your life depends on having an orgasm in five minutes. Who do you fantasize about? What do you imagine doing that will guarantee an orgasm?

The chances are high that this is a very secret fantasy. Most of us don't go around broadcasting our masturbation fantasies to our friends and relatives. However, even if you were to share one of your sexual fantasies with someone, you probably wouldn't share your primary fantasy. These fantasies tend to be somewhat mysterious. They excite us for reasons we don't fully understand. They often evoke a mixture of pleasure, confusion, and even shame. To help you get the most out of this chapter, I want you to set aside your inner judge or censor and use the emotion, power, and activity rating bars to describe your primary sexual fantasy.

I've asked hundreds of men and women to do this exercise.[30] I've also analyzed the written descriptions of their fantasies to identify the most commonly mentioned characters, settings, and activities. Then I presented these names and phrases to a new set of men and women, who then rated them separately on each of the emotion, power, and activity dimensions.

The results of these studies are mapped out in Figures 1 through 5. We'll look at each of these exercises to get a sense of the variety and scope of most men and women's fantasies. I'll ask you to circle your favorite characters, settings, and activities as well, so we can determine whether your fantasy preferences tend to cluster in particular sexual zones or if they fit a consistent pattern.

Who Is Your Ideal Fantasy Partner?

Let's start with who you find most appealing as a fantasy sexual partner. Exercise 1 maps out the most common fantasy men, and Exercise 2 presents the most popular fantasy women. These are occupations, personas, and archetypes that describe the type of person you would cast as the leading man or lady in your favorite sexual fantasy. If the character received a positive emotional rating in my studies, it's listed in the upper half of the page. Characters in the lower half are associated with a negative emotional tone and words such as *dark*, *dirty*, and *sinful*.

The diagrams also map out the average rating the characters received on both the power continuum (weak to strong) and the activity continuum (slow to fast). Characters in the *upper right* quadrant, for example, were seen (on average) as being both *fast* and *strong*.

Let's start by looking at how women rated their fantasy men. Characters with positive emotional associations who are seen as strong and active include a businessman, a pilot, a marine, and a star athlete. Examples from the negative or dark emotional continuum that are also fast and strong include a burglar, a gangster, and a boxer.

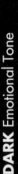

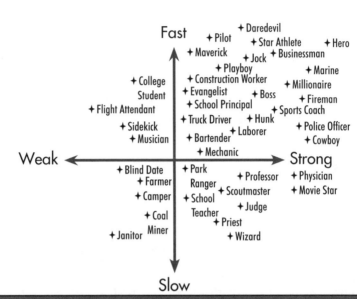

Exercise 1: Fantasy Men—Circle your fantasy lover.

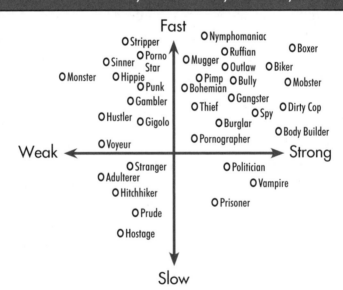

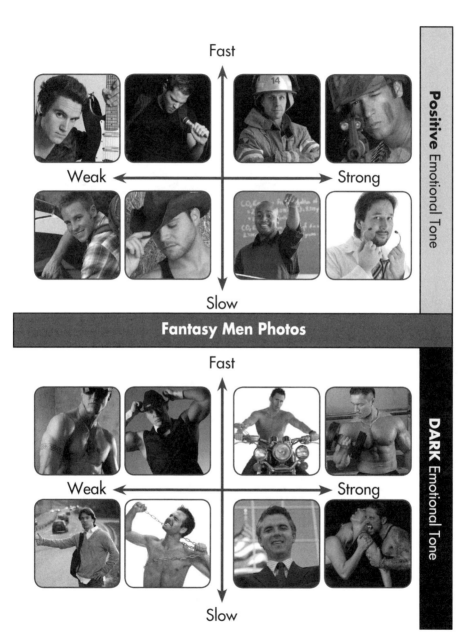

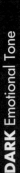

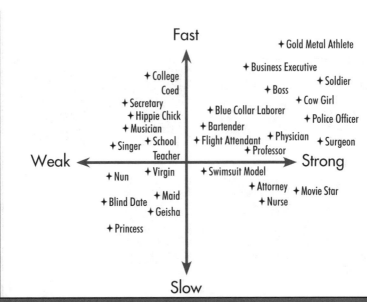

Positive Emotional Tone

Fast

+ Gold Metal Athlete

+ Business Executive

+ College Coed

+ Boss

+ Soldier

+ Secretary

+ Cow Girl

+ Hippie Chick

+ Blue Collar Laborer

+ Police Officer

+ Musician

+ Bartender

+ Singer + School Teacher

+ Flight Attendant + Physician + Surgeon

+ Professor

Weak ←——————————→ Strong

+ Swimsuit Model

+ Nun + Virgin

+ Blind Date + Maid

+ Attorney + Movie Star

+ Nurse

+ Geisha

+ Princess

Slow

Exercise 2: Fantasy Women—Circle your fantasy lover.

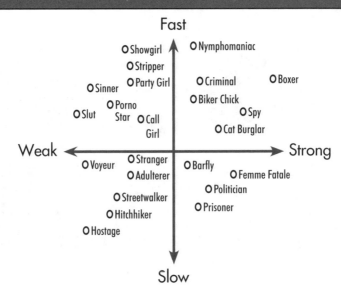

DARK Emotional Tone

Fast

O Showgirl O Nymphomaniac

O Stripper

O Sinner O Party Girl

O Criminal O Boxer

O Biker Chick

O Slut O Porno Star O Call Girl

O Spy

O Cat Burglar

Weak ←——————————→ Strong

O Voyeur O Stranger

O Adulterer

O Barfly

O Femme Fatale

O Politician

O Streetwalker

O Prisoner

O Hitchhiker

O Hostage

Slow

Fast

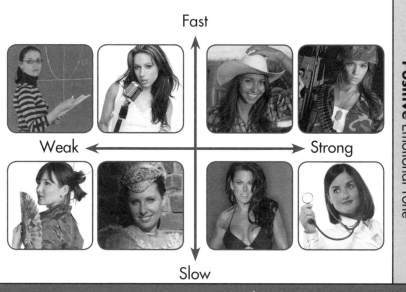

Weak ← → Strong

Slow

Positive Emotional Tone

Fantasy Women Photos

Fast

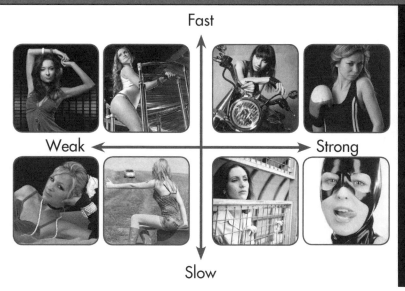

Weak ← → Strong

Slow

DARK Emotional Tone

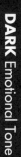

Fantasy men with opposite power and activity ratings, in the *lower left* quadrant, were viewed as *weak* and *slow*. Examples include a farmer and a camper in the positive emotional zone, and a stranger, a hitchhiker, and a hostage in the negative emotional zone.

As you can see, most of the fantasy men fall into the fast-strong quadrants. Still, women described fantasies with men in all eight quadrants, which suggests that every combination of emotion, power, and activity is potentially sexually exciting.

Exercise 2 presents the most commonly mentioned female fantasy characters, occupations, and archetypes, using the same framework. Fantasy women include a police officer and a cowgirl in the positive, strong, and fast quadrant. In the opposite quadrant, in the lower half of the page, one can find examples of negative, weak, and slow characters, including a streetwalker, a voyeur, and an adulterer.

In comparing the fantasy men versus fantasy women, two differences stand out. First, there are more male characters listed than female characters. In my research thus far, women offered a greater number of fantasy characters than did men.

Second, you may notice that most of the fantasy men are clustered in the strong and fast quadrants, while the female characters appear more evenly spread across the quadrants. Thus, while men offered a smaller *number* of female characters, they offered a wider *variety* of characters in terms of how they viewed their sexual power and activity levels.

Take a moment and circle the characters that *you* find most appealing. (Yes, if you bought the book, you can write in it.) Which characters have been in your fantasies? Which ones do you think you would enjoy fantasizing about?

You'll notice that I also included photo examples for each of the fantasy quadrants. Circle the photos you find most enticing. I believe your visual preferences are at least as effective as your verbal preferences in offering a window into your sexual tastes.

What Is Your Ideal Fantasy Setting?

Now that we've cast a leading man or lady for your sexual fantasy, we need to choose a sexy location. Exercise 3 presents the most common fantasy settings, divided into ones with a positive emotional tone in the upper half and ones with a dark emotional tone in the lower half.

It may seem odd to think of settings as being fast or weak. However, people tend to rate these settings in similar ways, and the resulting clusters have a certain logic. It makes sense that someone who fantasizes about having sex on an airplane, for example, might also fantasize about sex in an elevator; both are positive, strong, and fast. It makes sense that someone with a dark fantasy about having sex at a cheap motel might also fantasize about sex at an adult bookstore; both are dark, weak, and slow.

The settings in each of the quadrants also bring to mind very different scenarios, emotions, and types of sex. A fantasy that involves sex at a bed-and-breakfast, for example, will likely be very different from a fantasy that involves sex in the back of a police squad car.

It's time again to circle the names and photos of settings that you find most appealing. Have you fantasized about sex in any of these settings? Which settings inspire the most exciting sexual fantasies for you?

What Is Your Fantasy Role and Your Partner's Role?

We've cast your fantasy partner. He or she may be gentle and kind or nasty and dangerous. We've chosen a setting for the fantasy. It may be somewhere nice and fun or somewhere dark and gritty. Now we can get down to business. What do you do in your fantasy? What does your fantasy partner do? Together, what kind of sexual dynamic do you create?

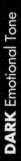

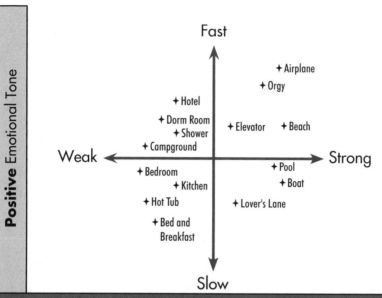

Positive Emotional Tone

Fast

+ Airplane
+ Orgy

+ Hotel
+ Dorm Room
+ Shower
+ Elevator   + Beach
+ Campground

Weak ←——————————→ Strong

+ Bedroom
+ Pool
+ Kitchen
+ Boat
+ Hot Tub
+ Lover's Lane
+ Bed and
Breakfast

Slow

Exercise 3: Fantasy Setting—Circle your ideal place for sex.

DARK Emotional Tone

Fast

○ Night Club
○ Amusement Park
○ Brothel
○ Military Boot Camp
○ Strip Club
○ Gymnasium
○ Cheap Motel
○ Sex Club   ○ Police Squad Car
○ Adult
○ Locker Room
Bookstore
○ Warehouse

Weak ←——————————→ Strong

○ Back of Car
○ Cave
○ Office
○ Alley ○ Prison
○ Public Restroom
○ Movie
Theatre
○ Church

Slow

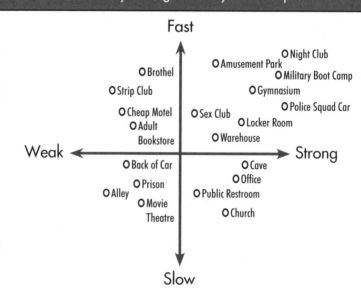

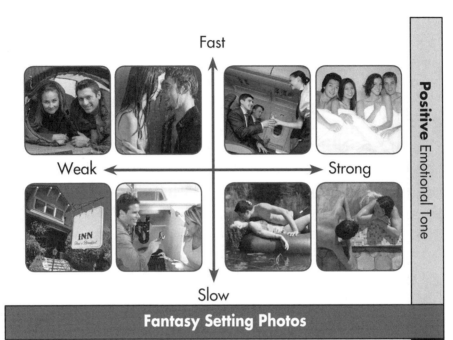

Fantasy Setting Photos

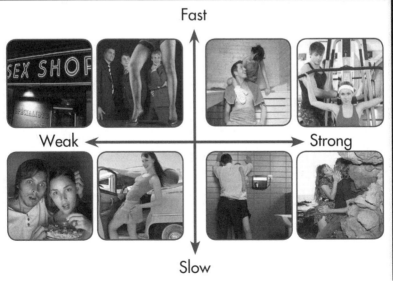

On opposing pages, Exercise 4 and Exercise 5 present a variety of activities for you and your ideal partner. The activities are positioned according to how most men and women see them in terms of their emotional tone, activity level, and power. Kissing, flirting, and undressing, for example, are seen as positive, strong, and fast things to do, while submitting and obeying are dark, weak, and slow activities.

Take a moment to circle what you would like to happen in your ideal fantasy.

When I've asked men and women to do this exercise, their choices tended to fit into one of three patterns. The first and most common pattern is to pick activities for you and your partner that are in the same emotional zone and usually in similar power and activity quadrants. If you like to kiss, snuggle, and make love in your fantasies, you probably want a partner who does the same.

The second pattern is to stay in the same emotional zone but put your actions in one quadrant and put your partner's in another. If you want to be positive, weak, and slow (for example, relax, surrender, be pleased orally), then you may want a partner who is positive, strong, and fast (for example, flirts, excites, pleases orally). Opposing quadrants often complement each other in fantasies.

The third pattern is to put your actions in one emotional zone and your partner's actions in the other emotional zone. You may want to play a positive role with a dark emotional partner, for example, and fantasize about surrendering, adoring, and moaning with pleasure while your partner plays rough, talks dirty, and ravishes you. Alternatively, you may want to play the dark role in your fantasy with a partner who is innocent and pure.

Where Is Your Sexual Fantasy Comfort Zone?

Take a moment to flip through the choices you've made for your favorite characters, settings, and activities. Do you see any commonalities or themes in your choices?

If most of your choices across the categories are in the upper half of the page, then your fantasies share a fun, flirtatious, and loving tone. If most of your choices are in the lower half of the page, then you are turned on by wild, dark, edgy, and dangerous sexual fantasies.

Obviously, if your choices center on a specific power and activity quadrant, this suggests you enjoy or are comfortable with specific kinds of sexual expression, but not others. I recommend you take note of the quadrants you avoided entirely. It is not uncommon, for example, for men to focus most of their choices in the strong quadrants and avoid the weak quadrants.

There's nothing wrong with enjoying one zone or a particular combination of zones. In Part 4 we'll look at ways to create new and exciting fantasies within your favorite and familiar sexual zones. Still, I believe there is also something to be gained by venturing outside of your comfort zone, especially if you avoid certain sexual zones out of fear or discomfort. In Part 4 we'll look at ways to use fantasy as a way to explore new sexual arenas and possibly uncover activities you might enjoy in real life.

If your choices are all over the page, then this suggests you have a wide-open fantasy landscape. If you want to dig a little deeper, I recommend you take a second pass and highlight a subset of characters, settings, and activities that you find exceptionally arousing.

People who circle lots of options are often highly sexual people, like the high sex drive and high adventurous types I described in Part 1. Their answer to every sexual question is "Yes, please!" But even if you enjoy all varieties of sex, chances are you like some options more than others. If you had to pick one or two sexual zones as most exciting and satisfying, which would you pick? Having a few core sexual fantasies in mind will be helpful in the next section as we explore the functions and motivations behind your sexual fantasies.

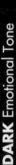

Positive Emotional Tone

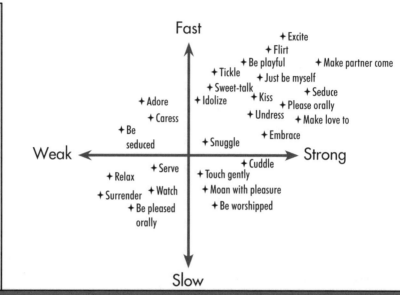

Fast

+ Excite
+ Flirt
+ Be playful   + Make partner come
+ Tickle   + Just be myself
+ Sweet-talk   + Seduce
+ Adore   + Idolize   + Kiss   + Please orally
+ Caress   + Undress   + Make love to
+ Be seduced   + Embrace
     + Snuggle
Weak ←――――――――――――――→ Strong
     + Cuddle
+ Relax   + Serve   + Touch gently
+ Surrender   + Watch   + Moan with pleasure
+ Be pleased orally   + Be worshipped

Slow

Exercise 4: Fantasy Actions—Circle what you want to do.

DARK Emotional Tone

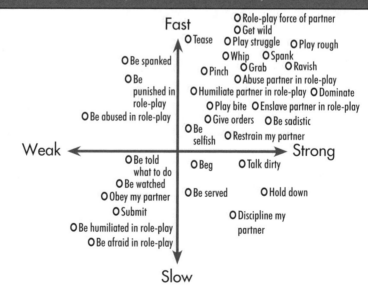

Fast

○ Role-play force of partner
○ Get wild
○ Tease   ○ Play struggle   ○ Play rough
○ Whip   ○ Spank
○ Be spanked   ○ Pinch   ○ Grab   ○ Ravish
○ Be punished in role-play   ○ Abuse partner in role-play
○ Humiliate partner in role-play   ○ Dominate
○ Be abused in role-play   ○ Play bite   ○ Enslave partner in role-play
○ Give orders   ○ Be sadistic
○ Be selfish   ○ Restrain my partner
Weak ←――――――――――――――→ Strong
○ Be told what to do   ○ Beg   ○ Talk dirty
○ Be watched
○ Obey my partner   ○ Be served   ○ Hold down
○ Submit
○ Be humiliated in role-play   ○ Discipline my partner
○ Be afraid in role-play

Slow

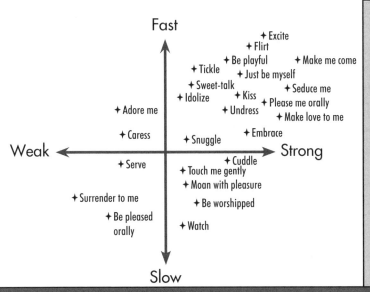

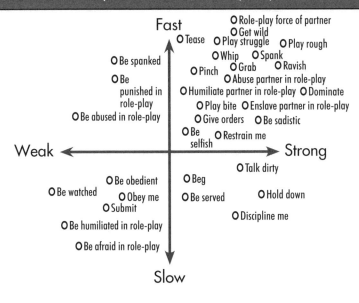

Exercise 5: Fantasy Actions—Circle what your partner should do.

Interpreting Your Sexual Fantasies

What Are the Most Common Wishes That Sexual Fantasies Fulfill?

Having studied thousands of fantasies and interviewed hundreds of men and women about the feelings of pleasure, confusion, and shame that often surround their fantasies, I've developed several hypotheses about why we fantasize about certain types of characters in particular types of situations. In the following sections, I present a framework that I believe can help you interpret your own fantasies and disentangle some of the mysteries of your inner sex life. We'll start by looking at some of the functions fantasies serve and explore some of the needs or wishes your fantasies may be fulfilling. Then we'll look at some of the fears and insecurities that get in the way of our fantasies and the three mental tricks our minds apply to get around these obstacles.

The oldest and most obvious explanation for why we have sexual fantasies is that they function as wish fulfillment. Sigmund Freud himself argued that sexual fantasies result from having our desires frustrated. He viewed them as desperate attempts to gratify forbidden wishes.

In modern society, the topics of sexual fantasies are not so much forbidden as they are denied by circumstances. As the Rolling Stones have taught us, there is usually a gap between what you want and what you get. Sexual fantasies are a convenient way to bridge that gap.

The wish fulfillment function of fantasies isn't limited to sex either. Fantasies can address many of our most basic human needs and wishes. They let us experience affection, control, and attention, even when we're alone. They give us the opportunity to have new experiences and feel new emotions without having to leave our apartments.

Let's take a look at five wishes or desires that sexual fantasies seem especially effective at satisfying:

1. *Sexual Variety.* As I mentioned in Chapter 2, fantasies offer a great way to explore a variety of sexual interests without having to have a sexual partner or a partner with the same interests. Especially for men and women with adventurous sexual tastes, fantasies offer a vehicle for imagining sex with different partners, exotic locations, and sex in every position in the *Kama Sutra.*

   Fantasies can also be a safe way to explore kinky activities and sex with dark emotional tones. This may include sexual activities that you may never try in real life, but are still exciting to fantasize about.

2. *Affection.* We are very social creatures. Humans actually need to be touched. A baby who is not touched or held will die just as reliably as if it were not fed. Adults may not need to be held (or burped) as much as babies, but there is evidence to suggest that humans are healthier and happier when they experience daily physical affection or even affection from a pet.

   What does this have to do with sexual fantasies you may ask? It turns out that both men and women often report fantasies that center on romance, affection, sensual touch, and kissing rather than intercourse or sex per se. I believe fantasies about being held and caressed are fulfilling a basic human need or wish for affection as much as a desire for sex.

3. *Control.* Fantasies often center on specific power dynamics (like being sexually dominant or submissive). It's possible that these fantasies give individuals a way to experience more (or less) control, depending on their life circumstances. If you feel like you have no control over your life, if your boss orders you around all day like a slave, then it

makes sense that a fantasy about having control sexually or otherwise would be pleasurable.

Conversely, if you feel burdened with responsibilities and choices all day (by your job, your family, and so forth), then it makes sense that a fantasy where you have no choice and no control would be a relief. Indeed, in my studies, this is a common explanation offered by men who enjoy being submissive to a dominatrix in fantasies or in role-play. They look to sex as a way to escape the burdens of responsibility.

4. *Creativity.* Next there's the wish or need to express creativity. I think creativity is both a gift and a burden. I lack any musical or artistic talent myself, but I've always been attracted to artists. One of the things I've noticed about artistic people is that they are never truly happy unless they are expressing their creativity. Yet, unfortunately, there are few opportunities to express creativity via our jobs and less time available to have creative hobbies.

Many men and women find an outlet for their creativity on the canvas of their fantasy life. In several of my fantasy studies, I've asked people to describe their favorite fantasy in writing. At first, I left room for about a paragraph. This was plenty of room for most people. However, I quickly learned that some people require much more space. I have received descriptions of fantasies that were basically abbreviated screenplays.

I suspect that these men and women enjoy imagining the characters, plots, and locations of their fantasies as much as the sexual part. I've had several men and women tell me that their fantasies were so real that they often felt like they were living a double life. Although this may seem a bit odd at first, maybe you've had similar feelings at times when you've been in the middle of reading a really good book or caught up in your favorite television series. Sometimes fictional characters in art or the ones we create in our mind can seem as real to us as any flesh-and-blood relationship.

Although I need to do a more extensive study of this phenomena, I have noticed that the people who write long fantasy descriptions are often the same ones who say they do not like or rarely watch pornography. Perhaps they are not interested in porn because they already have a rich fantasy life. It's also possible that the passive nature of watching porn robs them of the satisfaction of creating scenarios on their own.

5. *Attention.* Fantasies can fulfill not only present needs but also wishes and needs that arise from your past. Fantasies about being the center of sexual attention (like being eagerly serviced by a lover or being the focus of group sex) appear to be especially common among men and women who felt emotionally neglected in past relationships or in childhood.

Physical abuse has a profound impact on adults' internal and external sex lives. Parental neglect is also a form of abuse and can leave a lasting impact on a person's emotional needs and desire for recognition and attention. At least in fantasy, one can create a world where one is appreciated and never neglected.

Which of these wishes or needs resonate with you? Depending on the complexity of your fantasies, the simplest way to interpret them may be to recognize which combination of these needs motivates your inner sex life. To dig a little deeper, we'll need to look at the fears, frustrations, and insecurities that you've encountered in your external sex life and how your inner sex life deals with these.

How Do Fears and Insecurities Shape Your Fantasies?

All fantasies center in one way or another on something we want. I don't fantasize about eating brussels sprouts or one day owning a duplex in Trenton, New Jersey. No, I fantasize about eating ice cream and owning an island in Fiji.

In the previous section we looked at how fantasies can get straight to the point and imagine what you most want or need. However, sometimes your mind has to do some extra work. It has to create a fantasy context where your wishes and desires are possible.

Psychoanalyst Michael Bader explores this challenge in his book *Arousal: The Secret Logic of Sexual Fantasies.*[31] He argues that our minds create fantasies that eliminate the fears and frustrations that would prevent us from being aroused. Fantasies create an alternate universe where any barrier to sexual enjoyment is resolved or transformed.

His theory fits what cognitive scientists argue is the key function of imagination in general. Imagination is useful in part because it can obscure obstacles. It can make seemingly contradictory conditions coexist so we can imagine something that seems to be impossible.

Let's assume you want to have a fantasy about a person you find sexy or a sexual activity you find exciting or intriguing. Maybe you have a crush on a co-worker or someone hot at your gym. You sit back and start to imagine some sexual possibilities. However, just when you start to get aroused, some thought or fear pops into your mind and makes it impossible for you to get aroused or pursue the fantasy.

What are the fears, insecurities, or other mental turnoffs that can throw a cold towel on your sexy thoughts? In the studies I have done, here are the most common thoughts or fears that interfere with sexual arousal:

- "I'm not physically attractive or desirable."
- "I am incapable of seducing someone."

- "I won't be able to get aroused or stay aroused."
- "I can't please my partner sexually."
- "He or she will want to do something sexually that I don't like."
- "He or she won't like to have sex the way I enjoy it."
- "I'm too bored, sick, or tired to enjoy sex."
- "I feel guilty thinking about sex with anyone other than my spouse."

Do any of these thoughts sound familiar? Are there other thoughts or fears that pop into your mind whenever you want to explore sex in a fantasy or in real life? Many of these obstacles center on doubts and insecurities about one's value and capacity as a lover. Others refer to life experiences that blocked your desires or made you feel helpless.

These types of thoughts are the impetus for your mind's creative process. Your mind has to overcome or neutralize these obstacles in order for you to be aroused.

The way around these barriers is to remove you and your body from the sexual fantasy entirely. This is what happens when you watch pornography. As a voyeur, you're not expected to be part of the situation, be desired, or please a partner.

Fortunately, this is not the only option. Your mind has several creative tools it can use to neutralize your doubts, fears, and frustrations. In my research, I see three mental tricks pop up again and again.

Why Do Your Fantasies Travel through Time?

The first mental trick is time travel. The mind can create a fantasy that occurs in your past or in the future. If there is something about your present circumstance that makes it impossible for you to fulfill your sexual desires, then changing the time context can often resolve this.

If you want to fantasize about someone other than your current partner, perhaps it is more comfortable to imagine the scenario five or ten years ago, before you met your partner. If your current relationship is in trouble, perhaps it is easier to imagine feeling sexual in a not too distant future when you are single again. If you are depressed or unhappy with your life in general, it may be easier to imagine sex anywhere or at any time other than where you are right now.

Why Are You a Different Person in Your Fantasies?

Your mind's second creative trick is the ability to change who you are in your past, present, or future. This can include changing your age, weight, fitness, looks, or even your gender. If the fantasy is set in the past, your mind can transform you into the person you were at age eighteen or thirty or any age when you felt more at ease with yourself and sex.

Sometimes, self-transformation is a way to enjoy sexual variety. It's not uncommon for men and women to be curious about what sex would be like from the point of view of the opposite gender. Indeed, in my surveys, about one in three men and women say they have fantasized at least once about what sex would be like if they switched genders.

In most cases, however, the extent of self-transformation is a function of how dissatisfied one is with his or her current age or appearance. The more unattractive you feel, the more difficult it is to imagine being sexually desired. Indeed, the most common obstacle a fantasy must overcome is self-doubt and self-loathing associated with one's appearance and body image.

The mind can work around this obstacle by transporting you back to a time when you looked and felt sexy. Alternatively, you may feel more comfortable imagining sex at some point in the future, after you finish your diet or start going to the gym again.

Sometimes the transformations take place in the present and involve a change that makes you look and feel more attractive. If you are unhappy with your weight, your mind can trim off those extra pounds in an instant. Maybe it's easier for you to imagine having sex with the person you desire if you were blond, more handsome, taller, and so forth.

If you are really unhappy with who you are, it may be easier to imagine yourself as a different person entirely. Maybe it's easier to imagine having sex if you were your best friend or the sexy person at the gym whom everyone stares at or a popular movie star. Again, it's not uncommon for sexually adventurous individuals to imagine sex from different points of view just for the thrill of it. However, the focus here is on individuals who can only feel aroused if they change who they are.

Although physical appearance is the most common source of insecurity, it's not the only one. Men and women who feel socially awkward or shy may imagine being a person who is more confident and outgoing. A man embarrassed by erectile dysfunction may fantasize that he has the kind of sustained erection that the Viagra advertisements warn about. Unfortunately, there are many reasons a person may feel inadequate and unlovable. The ideal fantasy removes these imperfections or gives you new skills and attributes that make you desirable despite these limitations.

Why Is My Fantasy Lover Less (or More) Attractive Than Me?

The final creative trick in your mental toolbox is the ability to fashion a lover who makes you feel sexy. There are three main options. Your fantasy lover can be more attractive than you, equally attractive, or less attractive.

Chances are that you will want to create a fantasy lover who will find you attractive. If you transform your appearance in a fantasy (and become younger, thinner, taller, etc.), it's probably to reassure yourself that your fantasy lover will find you appealing. Alternatively, you can create a fantasy lover who is attracted to the current or real you. You can create a lover who, like Mark Darcy in the 2001 film *Bridget Jones's Diary,* thinks you are perfect "just the way you are."

The value of this admiration depends in part on the status or attractiveness of your fantasy lover. If you are fantasizing about a real or imagined person who is *more* physically attractive or more powerful, wealthy, or famous, then his or her attraction to you validates your appeal. This attractive person gives you permission to find yourself sexy and enjoy your fantasy sex.

Alternatively, you can fantasize about a lover who is *less* attractive or has *lower* status. This arrangement gives you a higher *relative* status; you are more attractive by comparison. In this fantasy, *you* are the pretty one. Perhaps he or she is much older, shorter, poorer, or has some other perceived disadvantage. Regardless, he or she is lucky to have sex with someone as hot and sophisticated as you, so you don't have to worry about those extra pounds or any other perceived imperfection.

Another variation on the status gap involves fantasies about lovers from different social classes or cultures. For the person who feels socially awkward, a fantasy about a lover who doesn't speak your language frees you to focus on a purely physical seduction. A full-figured woman, for example, may enjoy a fantasy about being in a foreign country where her body type is appreciated and her foreign status makes her a celebrity. Different cultures also bring different rules. A fantasy about a lover from a primitive culture, for example, frees you to imagine new sexual rules and alternative standards of beauty.

What Does the Situation or Setting Tell Me about My Fantasy?

Real life has a way of frustrating our desires. The person you dig doesn't dig you. The timing is off, or the timing was right, but you were clueless about it until a week later. You have amazing chemistry with someone, but one or both of you are in a committed relationship. One of the great things about fantasies is that they can cut through all these inconveniences.

Humans have been such a successful species in part because of our vivid imaginations. We can imagine ways around obstacles and see other possible ways to get what we want.[32] Let's look at several of the fantasies people described in my surveys and their own explanations for what inspired them. I have edited their descriptions and framed the explanations in terms of obstacles and fantasy solutions.

Obstacle	Fantasy Solution
I have great sexual chemistry with someone, but I can't explore a sexual relationship because we work together and he is in a committed relationship.	We are on a business trip, and the plane crashes, leaving us marooned on a deserted island, where we fall in love and have passionate sex.
I am attracted to someone who is much younger. I can't pursue a relationship with him due to our age difference.	In my fantasy, I turn back the clock and am now his age. He is very attracted to me as I looked back then and picks me up at a bar.
Several years ago I was at a party, hanging out with someone I had a big crush on. I had the perfect opportunity to finally connect with her, but I misread the signals and didn't act on it. Now it's too late, but I look back and wish things had gone differently.	I have two fantasies about her. In one, I am at that party and she is sending me great signals, but this time I recognize the cues and act on them, and we end up going to my place and having wild sex. In another fantasy, I am at a similar party in the future with a different person, but I act on the situation in a smoother way.
I am attracted to a woman who doesn't really see me as a real man in a sexual way.	I have a fantasy where I walk around a corner and find she is being mugged. I jump in and save her. She thanks me for rescuing her, and we end up having sex.

Obstacle	Fantasy Solution
I am attracted to a man I work with, but I don't think he even knows my name.	The two of us get stuck in an elevator and have a chance to talk. It's hot in the elevator, so we end up taking off some of our clothes, and one thing leads to another.
I am in love with a close friend who doesn't love me in that way.	In my fantasy, my friend is in an accident, and I have to nurse him back to health. Then a romance blossoms.
I split up with my fiancé a couple of years ago. We had great sex but were not compatible otherwise.	I often fantasize about having sex with her or remember specific, really great evenings we spent together.
I would never cheat on my wife by having an ongoing affair. But I would like to have a one-time sexual fling with someone.	I fantasize about picking up a hitchhiker. We have sex in the back of the car. I drop her off somewhere, and we never see each other again.
I had a very strict upbringing. Sex has always involved a lot of rules.	I fantasize I'm on vacation and get lost in the jungle. I am rescued by a primitive tribe that is very open sexually. I have sex with many of the men and women.
I am usually too tired from long hours at work and then taking care of my family when I get home.	I fantasize about being on spring break back when I was in college. I have tons of energy. My friends and I act wild and crazy and have lots of fun sex.

In each of these fantasies, the individual found a way to remove a situational obstacle and rearrange his or her circumstances. In several cases, time travel or an orchestrated tragedy made an impossible romance possible. In other cases, the individuals used fantasies as a way to cope with major regrets and disappointments.

How Do Stereotypic Beliefs about Women Shape Men's Fantasies?

Other major themes that pop up again and again in sexual fantasies are our attitudes and beliefs about sex and gender. We saw in Part 2 how stereotypical beliefs about gender can interfere with relationships and our interpersonal sex life. In our inner sex lives, our fantasies often have to find ways to neutralize our fears and rigid beliefs about gender.

Often the fantasy solution is to go to the opposite extreme. If a man believes that women don't like sex, for example, he fantasizes about women who are nymphomaniacs. This is definitely a theme that runs through most pornography.

In my research, several other stereotypical beliefs about women come up again and again and appear to be managed via fantasies in similar ways. Here are the six most common gender beliefs and the ways many men address them in their fantasies.

Stereotypic Beliefs about Women	Fantasy Solution
Women don't like sex.	Women in his fantasies love sex. They are very vocal about their enthusiasm for and enjoyment of everything he does sexually.
Women are impossible to satisfy sexually.	Women in his fantasies tell him what to do, so he is sure to satisfy his partner. He imagines a woman who is sexually selfish so that he does not have to worry about pleasing her.

Stereotypic Beliefs about Women	Fantasy Solution
Women are too busy to be nurturing and loving.	He is the center of attention in his fantasies. He is often surrounded by several women who are totally focused on pleasing him. Women in subservient but caring roles, such as geishas, are popular fantasy archetypes.
Women are delicate and are easily hurt.	He fantasizes about women who are powerful and strong. Thus he does not have to worry about hurting them. Women police officers, soldiers, and Amazons are common fantasy archetypes.
Women have to be respected and treated like ladies, not objects.	He fantasizes about women from lower social classes and different cultures. He is not expected to treat these women as ladies. Street prostitutes, criminals, and "trashy" women are examples of fantasy archetypes.
Women are only attracted to strong and tough men.	He fantasizes about weak and fragile women. Their vulnerability makes him stronger by comparison. Fantasies about rescuing women are common.

How Do Stereotypic Beliefs about Men Shape Women's Fantasies?

A common fantasy theme among heterosexual women is the stereotypic belief that "real" men are tough and strong. Indeed, the most common characters in women's fantasies are in the upper right quadrant of the plots (fast and strong) in Exercise 1. Fantasies about men in blue-collar professions (such as auto mechanics, plumbers, and firemen) are popular examples of this stereotype.

Yet women's fantasies often transform these characters into having both masculine and feminine qualities. For example, she may fantasize about a strong fireman who rescues her, but then he becomes a tender and gentle lover when they have sex.

Understanding Violent Fantasies

Is Violence an Intrinsic Part of Sex?

My survey of sexual fantasies confirmed what earlier studies had observed: a large number of sexual fantasies contain imagery and scenarios involving force, violence, or humiliation.[33] About one in three sexual fantasies involve masochistic themes, including being tied up, forced to do things, spanked, and so forth.

Freud and others since him have observed that sex often contains hostile or aggressive actions, and that for some people, arousal depends on these elements. They argue that sex allows us to release both our erotic and aggressive urges at the same time.[34]

I personally do not buy into the argument that humans are naturally turned on sexually by the combination of sex and violence. An alternative explanation for the same phenomena is that both sex and violence are physiologically arousing, and it is not always easy to distinguish between different forms of arousal.

If you are drawn to sexual fantasies that are both *fast* and *strong*, then it is understandable that excitement in any form can be a bridge to sexual arousal.[35] Even a ride on a roller coaster will probably make you horny. However, this does not imply that you have "roller coaster urges" that have to be satisfied as part of sex.

Indeed, if you prefer sex that is both *slow* and *weak*, then violence is probably a total turnoff for you. A roller-coaster ride or other fast and strong experiences would probably reduce your interest in sex (and increase your desire to throw up).

Nevertheless, if violence is not a necessary or intrinsic part of sex, why do violent themes pop up so frequently in our sexual fantasies? To apply the framework I described in the previous section, we would have to work backwards. First, we have to determine who is enacting the violence. If it is the fantasy partner, then we have to ask: what perceived obstacle or barrier does having an abusive partner resolve? If you are the source of the violence, we have to ask: how does portraying your lover as a victim of your force or abuse resolve a perceived obstacle to enjoying sex? In the next two sections, I propose possible answers to each of these questions.

Does Physical and Sexual Abuse Explain Violent Fantasies?

One way violence comes to inhabit our inner sex life is via the experience of physical or sexual abuse in childhood. British psychoanalyst Brett Kahr (author of *Who's Been Sleeping in Your Head?*) has studied sexual fantasies in both clinical settings and the general population.[36] In addition to the lasting impact of parental and family abuse, he also describes how mistreatment by peers, especially incidents of bodily humiliation and cruelty, can shape adult fantasies.

Kahr points out that some abused individuals create adult sexual fantasies that are direct repetitions of actual events in childhood. He argues that for these individuals the sexual fantasy reduces the distress of their memories by eroticizing them. A painful childhood experience is transformed into a pleasurable adult experience.

More commonly, however, adults who were abused as children base some aspects of their fantasies on childhood experiences, but they disguise or transform them in some way. Individuals often switch roles in their fantasies, for example, and identify with the aggressor rather than the recipient of abuse.

So I believe violent real-life experiences probably do play a role in shaping many individuals' violent sexual fantasies. Still, sadistic and masochistic fantasies are so widespread and popular that I doubt they can all be traced to abusive histories. So let's consider some other possible explanations.

What Is the Appeal of Fantasies about Being Forced?

In my surveys, both men and women commonly report fantasies about being forced to have sex or perform specific sexual acts. Almost without exception, these individuals always add (often in capital letters) that this is *not* something they want to occur in reality. Imagining something is definitely not the same as wanting it.

They understand, as I'm sure you understand, that force and abuse are never acceptable parts of sex. Indeed, they are serious crimes that inflict serious and lasting harm on their victims.

I think it's important to note that fantasies about force, even violent force, usually have an unreal or dreamlike quality. They do not elicit feelings of actual fear or pain. Indeed, the reason we have fantasies is to feel pleasure and sexual arousal. So we have to ask: How does a fantasy about force make it easier for some individuals to experience pleasure? What obstacle does this fantasy resolve or work around?

One interpretation is that fantasies about being forced free people from feeling any responsibility for choosing a forbidden sexual desire. If fantasizing about someone other than your current partner makes you feel guilty, for example, perhaps it's easier to fantasize about being forced by a mysterious partner. Having a fantasy about force can free you from having to feel guilty about "choosing" to be unfaithful or finding someone other than your partner to be sexually desirable.

Fantasies about force can also open the door to exploring the wilder and nastier aspects of sex. It can give you a chance to explore dark fantasy characters (like burglars, strippers, or prisoners) and wilder sexual activities (like restraint, spanking, or rough play) without having to condone or accept this form of sexuality.

A somewhat different variation on force involves fantasies of being taken sexually. Many romance novels and more than a few movies portray a male character so overcome by desire that he ravishes a woman sexually. The scene is not rape per se, but it does involve dominant, assertive, or aggressive actions.

For example, in the 1981 movie *Body Heat*, William Hurt throws a chair through a glass door in order to reach a sultry Kathleen Turner. In scenes like these, aggressive sexual action is presented as a twisted form of flattery for the desired woman.

So it's easy to understand how a person who feels unattractive or undesirable can incorporate force into a fantasy as a means of validating his or her desirability. Not only is she attractive in the fantasy, she is *so* appealing that she overpowers him with her seductive charms, forcing him to lose all control and throw himself on her.

I am not endorsing this point of view. I am simply pointing out that this scenario has been widely promoted. So it's understandable that a number of men and women incorporate similar scenarios into their fantasies.

Why Do People Fantasize about Being the Aggressor?

In real life, rape is fundamentally an act of violence and control rather than sex. Among some men, fantasies about rape and sexual force are also essentially about hostility toward women. Nevertheless, according to Brett Kahr and Michael Bader, who have studied this topic in greater depth than I have and who've clinically interviewed hundreds of subjects, the vast majority of men with rape fantasies have no history of violence or aggression toward women. For most men, fantasies about force appear to serve some other creative function. Again, we have to work backwards and ask: what obstacle, fear, or insecurity does a fantasy about force resolve?

One explanation is that a fantasy about force allows the man to be sexually selfish and frees him from any responsibility to try to understand or satisfy his partner's needs. One of the most common insecurities and frustrations among men is their uncertainty about what women want sexually and how to please them. A man who fantasizes about being completely selfish sexually frees himself from having to worry about satisfying his partner.[37]

Although I have tried to maintain a nonjudgmental attitude in my research, I have to admit I struggle with the meaning and implications of fantasies about rape and abuse. For whatever reason, I am somewhat less concerned about fantasies involving being the *recipient* of force or abuse. In these fantasies, the individual is in control of *both* the actor and the recipient of abuse.

My primary concern is with the long-term psychological and interpersonal impact of entertaining fantasies that portray women as targets of hostility and violence. I should add that many of the men with these fantasies also worry about their meaning and try not to have them.

Can recognizing the doubts and insecurities behind violent fantasies weaken their hold on one's inner sex life? In psychotherapy, gaining insight into the source of obsessions and compulsions rarely has a magical effect. Nevertheless, it can be a step toward change. If you are troubled by violent fantasies, I hope that you can recognize that your inner sex life has chosen this as one way of dealing with your doubts and fears. It may have been an efficient and effective solution so far in your life, but it doesn't have to be the only solution.

Take a look at the other fantasy characters, settings, and actions you circled in the earlier exercises. Try to introduce some of these new fantasy characters and plot devices to address your sexual fears and insecurities. If you feel the only way to be aroused is to fantasize about violence, I believe you can at least expand your set of fantasy options and find nonviolent scenarios that are at least equally as pleasurable.

Chapter 10

Sexual Personas
Which Styles Fit with Your Own?

Bedroom Surprises

Why Do We Encounter Bedroom Surprises?

One of the surprising things about dating that no one ever prepares you for is that the person you meet and have dinner with is not always the same person you encounter when the lights go off in your bedroom.

Back when I wrote a dating advice column, I received a lot of letters about these "bedroom surprises." Some of them were good surprises. Julie in Santa Fe, New Mexico, had skirted around the invitations of a sweet, mild-mannered guy from work for over a year, because she thought he was a little too nice and a tad boring. However, the man she met when they finally got naked was an entirely different person. He was a noisy, energetic, and adventurous wild man in the sack. Their sexual chemistry was off the charts.

Some bedroom surprises are disappointments. Aaron in Albany,

New York, for example, wrote about a fun, energetic woman he dated for several months. They both loved adventure sports, liked mountain biking, and spent every weekend on the go, doing fun, new things. Aaron had intentionally delayed having sex, because he thought their connection could turn into something serious. He felt certain that the sexual chemistry would be there when they decided to take that step. However, it turned out their relationship totally fizzled when it became sexual. Even after a few nights of earnest efforts on both their parts, the two of them never seemed to click sexually. He was disappointed and confused because the energetic and vivacious woman he had been dating was totally missing in the bedroom. She was much more passive and conservative sexually than he had expected, and ultimately they called it quits.

Have you ever encountered a good or bad bedroom surprise? Have your lovers acted in ways that were consistent with their personality? Or has sex brought out new and interesting parts of their personality that you had not glimpsed before?

Do *you* surprise your partners sexually? Do you think, act, or feel like a different person when you're naked with someone? Are you cool and confident in public, but neurotic and insecure sexually? Or maybe you're like Superman and have to strip away your boring work costume to reveal the confident and powerful real you underneath.

The key to understanding these bedroom surprises and unlocking the mysteries of sexual chemistry lies in our ability to distinguish between our public personality and our sexual personality. We need to appreciate that sex brings out a very unique part of our identity. Sometimes this sexual side is consistent with a person's public face, but often sex brings out unique emotions, attitudes, and behaviors that don't show up in other contexts.

How Many Personalities Do You Have?

Back when I was in graduate school, the conventional wisdom was that each individual had *one* primary personality. Only actresses in Lifetime television movies had *multiple* personalities.

More recent theories have had to reconcile the fact that even normal men and women can act in very different ways, depending on the situation. You can be serious and analytical at work, but then you can be playful and silly when you meet your friends for a drink after work. You are still you in both situations, but different aspects of your personality are expressed depending on who you're with, what the rules are, and what's expected of you.

It turns out that Walt Whitman had it right when he said, "We contain multitudes."[38] We are collections of multiple selves.[39]

By the time you entered high school, you probably already had *at least* two distinct personalities. One was probably aligned with your *family*, and the other was probably shaped by your *friends.*

As an adult, you probably developed a distinct professional identity as well. Your job probably requires you to bring out certain parts of your personality and suppress others. If you work in retail, for example, you have to be outgoing, friendly, and polite and suppress parts of yourself that are impatient, disinterested, or sarcastic.

Depending on how many different hats you wear in your life (as an employee, boss, parent, sibling, friend, spouse, and so forth), you probably have at least six distinct selves that involve specific ways of thinking, acting, and feeling. In addition to these public faces, most of us also have at least one sexual persona that comes out when we connect with someone sexually.

Obviously, the framework I presented in Part 2 that boiled personalities into eight types is a simplified version of a much more complex phenomenon. In Chapter 3 I asked you to think about your general public persona, the face that you present to the outside world most of the time. We also explored which of the eight public personas you found most attractive and tended to be drawn to for dating or relationships. I still believe this shorthand way of viewing personality can be useful. It can help you to understand your own makeup and your unique strengths and challenges. As we saw in Chapter 3, if you're single, it can also help you anticipate the kinds of sex drives and sexual interests that tend to go with certain personality types.

But now it's time to get more specific and look at your unique sexual self and the part of your personality that comes out in intimate, sexual contexts. We may discover that your sexual persona is similar to your public persona, or it may be quite distinct from your public self and lead to occasional bedroom surprises. We may find that the sexual persona you find most attractive and compatible is similar to the external public persona you're drawn to, or you may be drawn to very different styles in and out of the bedroom.

They say that "consistency is the hobgoblin of little minds."[40] Having consistent public and sexual personas and being attracted to similar types in and out of the bedroom doesn't mean you have a little mind, but it definitely translates into having a simpler and more straightforward sex life. But if your public and sexual personas are not consistent, or you're drawn to complicated traits in and out of the bedroom, I doubt there is much you can do to change that. I doubt you can make yourself more internally consistent or change who and what you find attractive. If you're not consistent by nature, then you simply have to work harder to understand yourself, search more carefully for a compatible partner, and put more effort into creating an engaging long-term sexual connection with someone.

I wrote this chapter to help you on that journey. You'll identify your own sexual persona and the personas you are drawn to. We'll explore which sexual personas tend to click, and which tend to be on different sexual wavelengths. We'll see which sexual personas tend to have higher sex drives and more adventurous sexual tastes. This will set the stage for Part 4, where I'll describe strategies for finding a partner with a compatible sexual persona and what you can do to improve your connection if your styles don't automatically click.

What Is Your Sexual Persona?

What Factors Combine to Create Your Sexual Persona?

The foundation of your sexual persona is made up of the three core dimensions we reviewed in the previous chapters: emotional tone, power, and activity. In Chapter 9 we saw how these three dimensions combine as part of your *inner* sex life to create your ideal sexual fantasy zone. Now we're going to shift the focus to the real world and your interpersonal sex life.

Let's start by identifying the sexual persona that most closely fits your sexual energy and how you approach sex. Take a look at Exercise 1 (for women) or Exercise 2 (for men). I've written the questions in these exercises two ways so you can use them to identify your own sexual persona and the persona you find most attractive in a potential partner.

Let's start with describing your own personal style. Complete the exercise with the photos that match your gender. Based on what you learned in Chapter 6, would you say you approach sex with a dark, sinful, and nasty style or a positive, wholesome, and innocent style? Based on what you learned in Chapter 7, would you say you prefer to play a more gentle and submissive role or a more powerful and dominant role? Finally, based on what you learned in Chapter 8, would you say that the energy you bring to sex is slow and tender or fast and intense?

Your choices at these three branches in the chart will lead you to one of eight sexual personas. I've also included a set of adjectives to describe each style or persona at the bottom of the chart. So if you have trouble picking one direction or another in the chart, take a look at the words describing each persona and pick the set of words that comes closest to describing your typical or most natural approach to sex.

If you find your style could fit in more than one of these categories, make a note of this too. There's no rule that says you can have

Exercise 1: Women's Sexual Personas

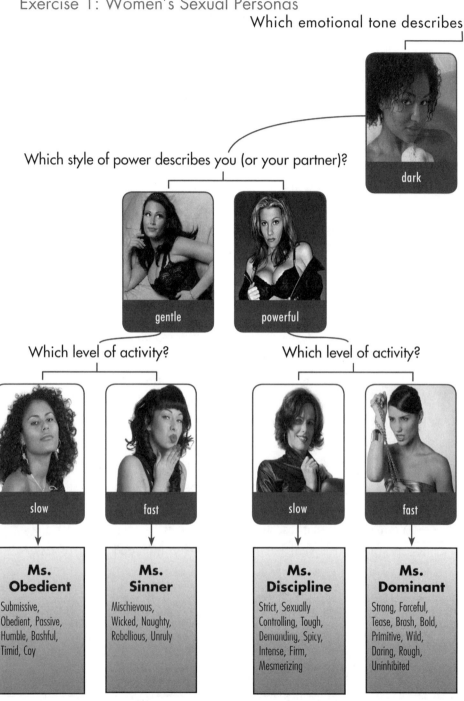

Which emotional tone describes

dark

Which style of power describes you (or your partner)?

gentle

powerful

Which level of activity?

Which level of activity?

slow

fast

slow

fast

Ms. Obedient

Submissive, Obedient, Passive, Humble, Bashful, Timid, Coy

Ms. Sinner

Mischievous, Wicked, Naughty, Rebellious, Unruly

Ms. Discipline

Strict, Sexually Controlling, Tough, Demanding, Spicy, Intense, Firm, Mesmerizing

Ms. Dominant

Strong, Forceful, Tease, Brash, Bold, Primitive, Wild, Daring, Rough, Uninhibited your (or your partner's) sexual style?

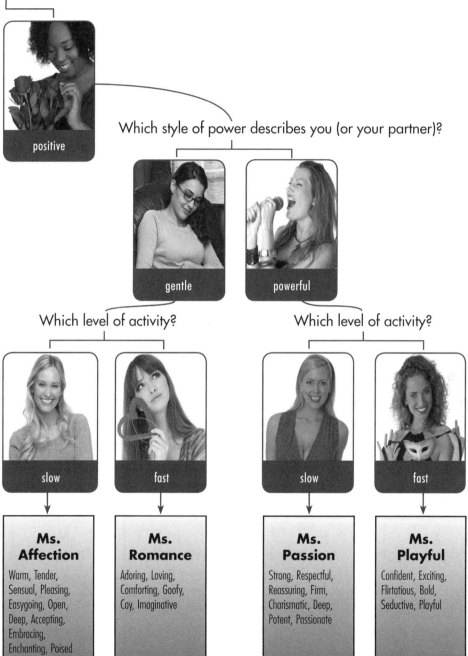

positive

Which style of power describes you (or your partner)?

gentle

powerful

Which level of activity?

Which level of activity?

slow

fast

slow

fast

**Ms.
Affection**

Warm, Tender,
Sensual, Pleasing,
Easygoing, Open,
Deep, Accepting,
Embracing,
Enchanting, Poised

**Ms.
Romance**

Adoring, Loving,
Comforting, Goofy,
Coy, Imaginative

**Ms.
Passion**

Strong, Respectful,
Reassuring, Firm,
Charismatic, Deep,
Potent, Passionate

**Ms.
Playful**

Confident, Exciting,
Flirtatious, Bold,
Seductive, Playful

Exercise 2: Men's Sexual Personas

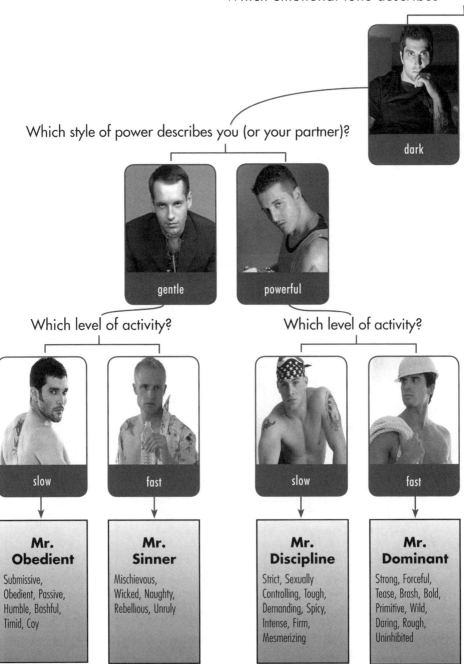

Which emotional tone describes

dark

Which style of power describes you (or your partner)?

gentle

powerful

Which level of activity?

Which level of activity?

slow

fast

slow

fast

Mr. Obedient

Submissive, Obedient, Passive, Humble, Bashful, Timid, Coy

Mr. Sinner

Mischievous, Wicked, Naughty, Rebellious, Unruly

Mr. Discipline

Strict, Sexually Controlling, Tough, Demanding, Spicy, Intense, Firm, Mesmerizing

Mr. Dominant

Strong, Forceful, Tease, Brash, Bold, Primitive, Wild, Daring, Rough, Uninhibited you (or your partner)?

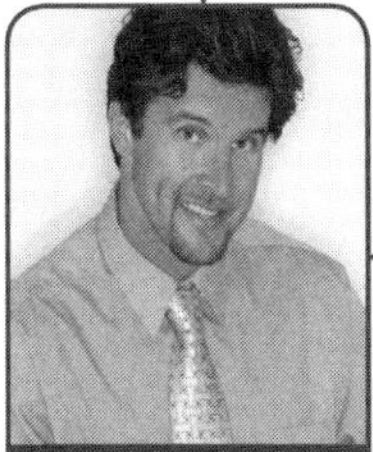

positive

Which style of power describes you (or your partner)?

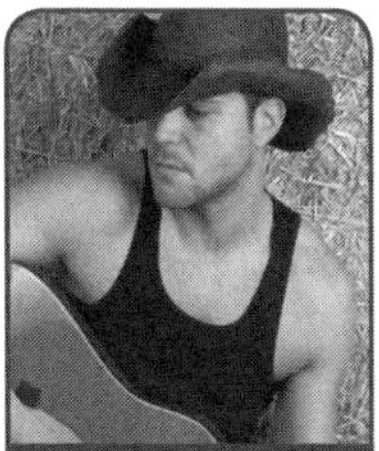

gentle

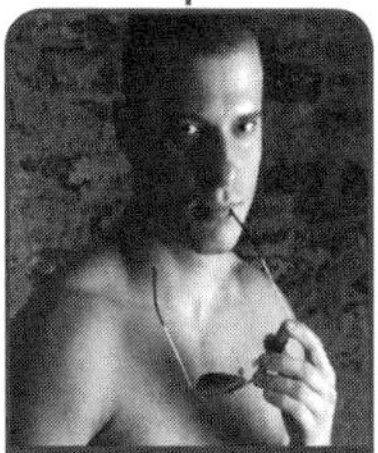

powerful

Which level of activity?

slow

fast

Which level of activity?

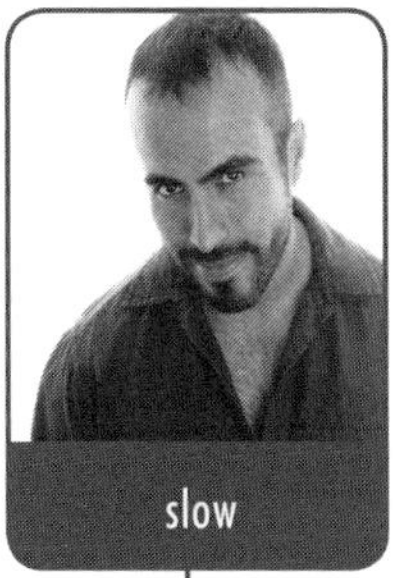

slow

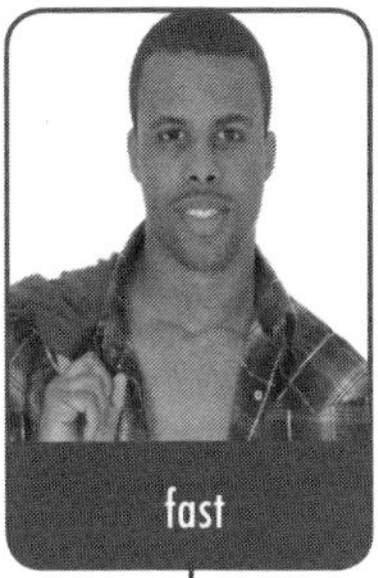

fast

Mr. Affection

Warm, Tender, Sensual, Easygoing, Open, Deep, Accepting, Embracing, Meek Enchanting, Poised

Mr. Romance

Adoring, Loving, Comforting, Goofy, Coy, Imaginative, Pleasing

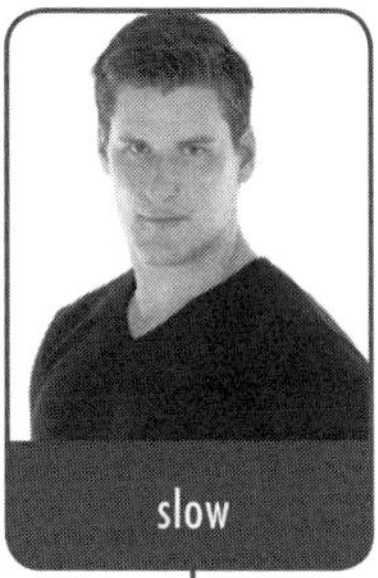

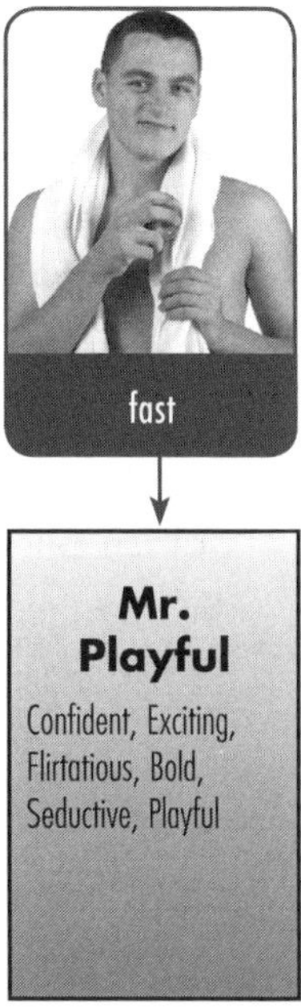

Mr. Passion

Strong, Respectful, Reassuring, Firm, Charismatic, Deep, Potent, Passionate

Mr. Playful

Confident, Exciting, Flirtatious, Bold, Seductive, Playful

only one style. You may have a versatile style and enjoy taking on different personas, depending on who you're with or what you're doing sexually. We talked a bit about versatility in Chapter 7 as it pertains to power dynamics, and we'll take a closer look at the implications of having multiple sexual personas in Chapter 11.

What Are the Most and Least Common Sexual Personas?

Based on research using these exercises, as well as studies with more in-depth inventories, I have estimated the proportion of men and women with each of the eight sexual personas.[41] You'll find these statistics in the first column of Figure 1 (for women) and Figure 2 (for men).

Among both men and women, more people identify with sexual personas with a positive emotional tone than a dark tone. In other words, when people describe their own sexual style, most people branch to the right of the chart and say they approach sex with a positive, wholesome, and innocent emotional tone. In fact, two out three men and women fit into one of the four sexual personas with a *positive* emotional tone.

The most common sexual persona among women, for example, is Ms. Romance; one in four women identify with this combination of positive emotions, gentleness, and fast intensity. The men are more equally divided among the positive emotional categories.

On the darker side of the spectrum, roughly one in ten men and women fall into each of the darker sexual personas. Ms. Sinner is the most common persona among women, and Mr. Sinner is the most common among men. For women, this is not that surprising, especially when you consider that Ms. Sinner is the darker emotional version of Ms. Romance, and they both share a gentle but active approach to sex. I was a bit more surprised with how common Mr. Sinner was among men. Contrary to what I expected, slightly more men prefer a submissive style than a dominant style.

Figure 1: Proportion of Women with Each Sexual Persona and Their Popularity

	% of Women	Men Who Find Her Sexy	Men Who Find Her Unappealing
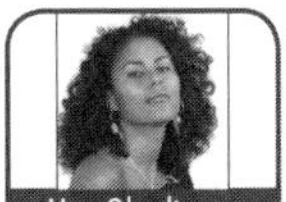 Ms. Obedient	9%	17% ✚✚	29% ⬇⬇⬇
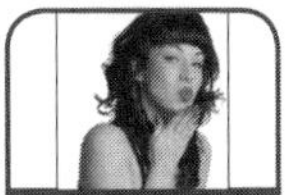 Ms. Sinner	14%	23% ✚✚	27% ⬇⬇⬇
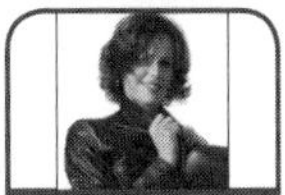 Ms. Discipline	6%	27% ✚✚✚	28% ⬇⬇⬇
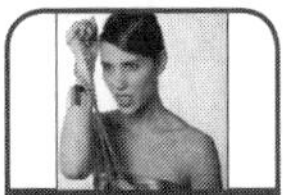 Ms. Dominant	8%	32% ✚✚✚	21% ⬇⬇
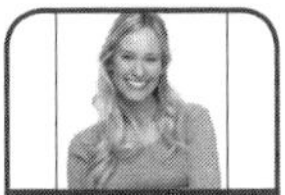 Ms. Affection	16%	31% ✚✚✚	28% ⬇⬇⬇
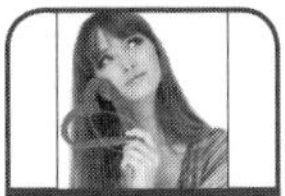 Ms. Romance	23%	57% ✚✚✚✚✚✚	13% ⬇
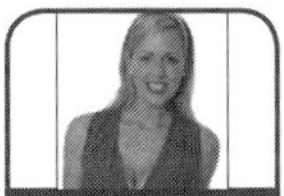 Ms. Passion	10%	38% ✚✚✚✚	21% ⬇⬇
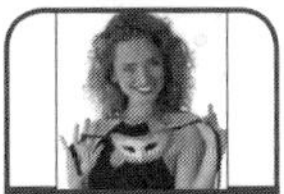 Ms. Playful	14%	62% ✚✚✚✚✚✚	21% ⬇⬇

✚ and ⬇ = Approximately 10%

Figure 2: Proportion of Men with Each Sexual Persona and Their Popularity

	% of Men	Women Who Find Him Sexy	Women Who Find Him Unappealing
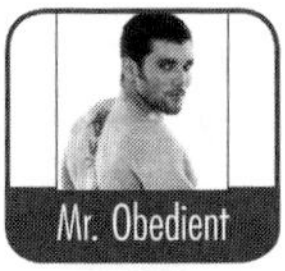 Mr. Obedient	10%	13% ✚	27% ↓↓↓
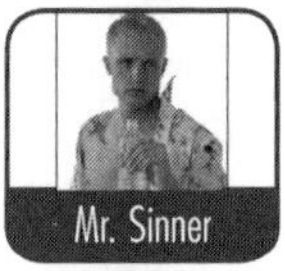 Mr. Sinner	12%	17% ✚✚	29% ↓↓↓
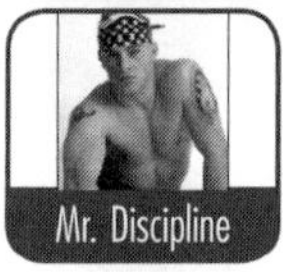 Mr. Discipline	7%	33% ✚✚✚	30% ↓↓↓
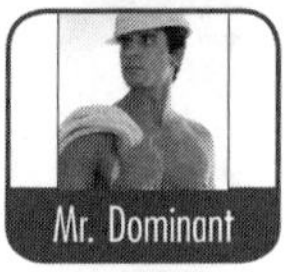 Mr. Dominant	8%	42% ✚✚✚✚	27% ↓↓↓
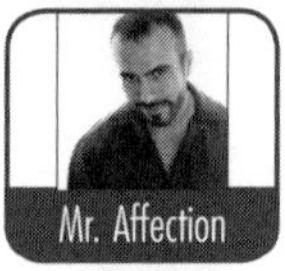 Mr. Affection	17%	52% ✚✚✚✚✚	23% ↓↓
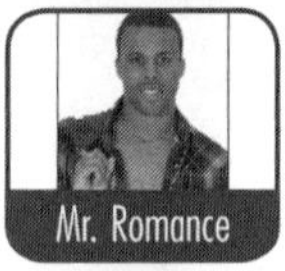 Mr. Romance	17%	61% ✚✚✚✚✚✚	18% ↓↓
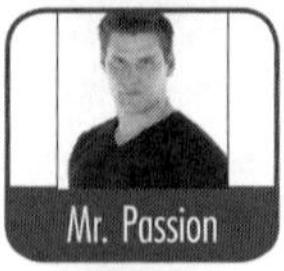 Mr. Passion	13%	33% ✚✚✚	27% ↓↓↓
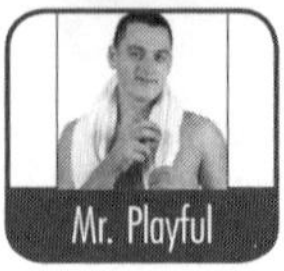 Mr. Playful	16%	61% ✚✚✚✚✚✚	22% ↓↓

✚ and ↓ = Approximately 10%

Why Are These Numbers Surprising and Important?

I'm fascinated by the distribution of men and women into the sexual persona categories for several reasons. First, there is so much secrecy surrounding sex that it's easy to feel that your particular approach to sex is odd or weird. My research suggests that there are sizable numbers of men and women in each of the sexual personas. Even an individual with the rarest style shares his or her approach with at least one in ten men and women.

The findings also challenge many gender stereotypes about sex and sexuality. Clearly, not all women have a wholesome and innocent approach to sex. The proportion of men and women who have a dark, sinful, and naughty approach to sex is very similar (about one in three). Most women have a gentler and more submissive sexual style, but at least one in three like to play a strong, forceful, and dominant role sexually. Fortunately, there are plenty of men who are looking for a dominant partner; almost half of all men prefer to play a gentler and more submissive sexual role.

Finally, these statistics are important and relevant for single men and women trying to find a compatible partner. As we'll see in Chapter 11, the popularity of your own sexual style and the percentage of men or women who fit in a category you find appealing translate into the odds of your finding a compatible partner. A man who is attracted to women with a wholesome and sensual approach to sex, for example, has a much better chance of finding a compatible partner than a man who is drawn to women with a darker, wilder, and more intense sexual style.

Are Your Public and Sexual Personas Consistent?

There are no simple formulas for comparing your public self with your private, sexual self. You could argue that this is a case of comparing apples and oranges. However, there must be some commonalities in style and energy that come across in public and in private.

If not, we couldn't pinpoint times when the two match up or when good or bad bedroom surprises occur.

To compare the two aspects of personality, we need to put both sets of personas in the same emotional tone, power, and activity framework. To graphically map this out, I borrowed the same grid we used in Chapter 9 to look at sexual fantasies, with the upper half showing personas with positive emotional associations and the lower half showing personas with darker emotional links.

Exercise 3 presents both sets of personas on opposite sides of the page using this grid. The left side of the page recaps the breakout of the eight sexual personas, with one style in each quadrant. So, for example, you will find Mr. and Ms. Playful in the positive, strong, and fast quadrant, while Mr. and Ms. Obedient are in the dark, weak, and slow quadrant.

The right side of the page shows the approximate placement of each public persona on the same dimensions. As you'll recall, I derived the public personas using traditional personality dimensions (the so-called Big 5), but the adjectives that describe each type can also be rated using the emotion, power, and activity dimensions. For example, most men and women rated the adjectives associated with Mr. and Ms. Grounded (upbeat, helpful, and supportive) as positive, strong, and fast.

As you can see, most of the adjectives that describe the public personas are associated with positive emotions. Only two of the personas (Adventurer and Rebel) have qualities with darker emotional associations (a risk taker, shrewd, and rebellious).

You'll also notice that some of the public personas are grouped in the same quadrant, which means they are similar on these underlying dimensions. Both the Shy and Nice personas, for example, share positive, weak, and slow qualities.

So your task in Exercise 3 is to put a check beside the sexual persona (or personas) that describe your sexual style, and then put a check beside the public persona (or personas) that best describe your public personality. If these two sides of your personality are consistent, then the check marks on both sides of the page should be in the same quadrants of the grid. The Faithful public personality, for example, is similar to the Romance sexual style. It would make sense that a person with a patient, caring, and friendly public personality would approach sex with an adoring, loving, and comforting style.

If the checks on each side of the page are in different quadrants, then your personality is more complex and may surprise your lovers. Earlier I described how Aaron (from Albany, New York) was dating a woman whose public personality fit Ms. Adventure. She was confident, spontaneous, energetic, and a thrill seeker. He expected her sexual style would be wild, daring, and uninhibited, like Ms. Dominant. However, she turned out to have a sexual style more like Ms. Affection that was slow, easygoing, and accepting.

The further apart in the grid your checks are, the more surprising and contrasting your two personas are. If your public personality fits the Rebel or Adventure type, for example, then most lovers are going to expect you to be an assertive and forceful lover who likes naughty and sinful sex.

As you'll see in Chapter 11, there is a trend toward consistency, especially for some of the personas and for certain broad underlying dimensions. Men and women with a Shy persona, for example, typically have a sexual persona that is slow in activity (like Mr. or Ms. Obedient, Sinner, Affection, or Romance). So there tends to be consistency in the speed, intensity, and movement associated with a Shy person's style both in and out of the bedroom.

In Part 4 we'll look at ways to communicate the consistent and inconsistent parts of your personality with potential partners. We'll also look at ways to embrace and enjoy your sexual style, regardless of how complex your traits are in and out of the bedroom.

Exercise 3: Compare Your Sexual and Public Personas

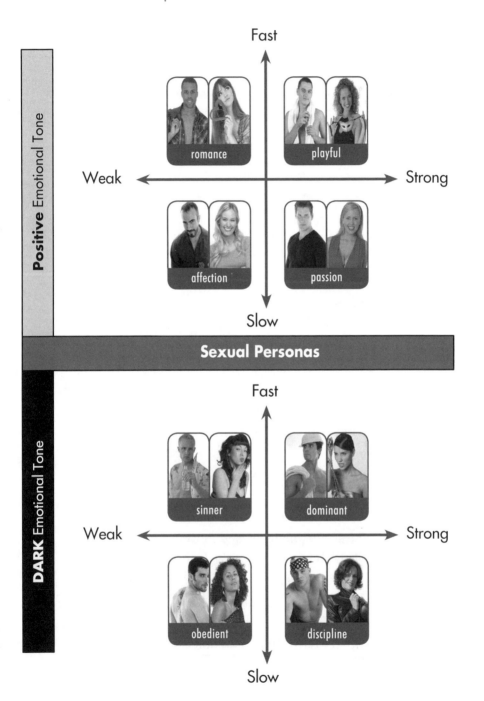

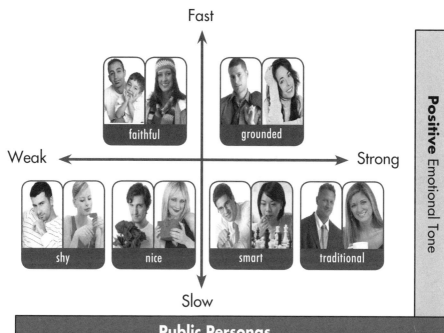

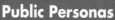

Public Personas

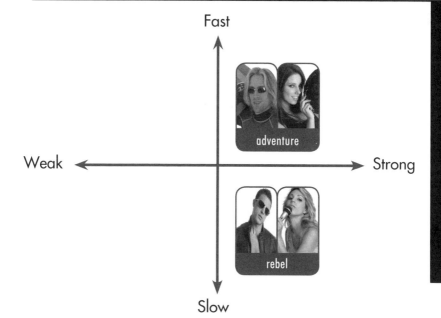

Which Sexual Personas Are You Drawn To?

Which Styles in Which Combinations Turn You On?

Now let's identify the sexual persona or personas you find most appealing. If you're single, you have a relatively easy task. Think of your ideal sexual partner. Then go through either Exercise 1 or Exercise 2 and pick the style you're drawn to. In most cases, people are drawn to partners who approach sex with a similar emotional tone, but this is not written in stone. It's not uncommon, for example, to find a person who has a dark and naughty approach to sex who is attracted to partners with a more wholesome or innocent sexual style.

On the power dimension, you may be drawn to partners with a similar style, or you may want a partner who complements or contrasts with your approach. If you tend to be more dominant, for example, you may want a partner who'll let you take the lead sexually.

People also tend to be drawn to partners with similar activity styles, but this is also not a firm rule. There are plenty of men and women with slow and tender styles who prefer a more active and intense lover and vice versa.

Regardless, pick the branches in the chart that match the style you are usually drawn to and make note of your preferred or ideal sexual persona. You can also refer to the adjectives that describe each style to help narrow down your favorite persona. If you find multiple styles appealing, that's good too, but for the purposes of this chapter try to pick one favorite or preferred persona.

If you are currently in a relationship, I recommend you go through the exercises two different ways. First, make the choices while thinking of your current partner and how he or she tends to approach sex. Then take a step back and think of your ideal partner or the type of partner you would be drawn to if you were single again. If you end up picking the same sexual persona both times, then you're lucky. Your current partner already embodies the sexual persona you are drawn to. If not, then things get a bit more complicated, and we'll need to look at strategies for connecting with your partner in new ways. That's the focus of Chapter 12. For now, let's take a closer look at which sexual personas are most and least popular and whether your tastes are similar to other men and women or rare.

Which Sexual Personas Are Most (and Least) Popular?

Go back and take a look at Figure 1 and Figure 2 to find the percentage of men and women who find each sexual persona attractive, as well as the percentage who finds the type unappealing.[42] In this research, I allowed people to pick multiple personas that they found appealing and multiple ones that they were definitely not interested in. Be sure to check out the popularity of your own sexual persona and the popularity of the sexual persona of your ideal or existing partner.

If you compare the two figures, you'll see that the most and least popular personas are very similar among both men and women. For both genders, Mr. and Ms. Romance and Mr. and Ms. Playful stand out as the most popular personas; two out of three adults find these styles attractive. Among the male personas, Mr. Affection is also very popular; half of all women find this style attractive. Most of the other personas are popular with about one in three men and women. So each sexual persona has a sizable target audience that appreciates their sexual style.

The *least* popular sexual personas for men and women are the two types with a dark emotional tone and low power (Obedient and Sinner). About one in three men and women find these personas unattractive or unappealing. These strong negative reactions reflect the fact that most men and women are less attracted to darker sexual styles. More passive or submissive styles are also somewhat less popular. Still, every sexual persona has its fans and its detractors. If you were just connecting with people at random, you'd only expect about one in three lovers would be totally turned on by your sexual style, and one in three would be turned off by your style. These aren't great odds. But if you've ever been frustrated by the hit-and-miss nature of sexual chemistry, these numbers should validate your experiences, if nothing else. Ideally, you want to stop dating at random and improve your odds by finding a partner whose style will mesh with your own. Let's look at how each of the styles fits with the other styles.

Which Sexual Personas Fit and Which Ones Clash?

To summarize the likely fit (or lack of fit) between each of the sexual personas, I created a table with the women's personas as rows and the men's personas as columns. This megatable is listed as Exercise 4. Start by finding your sexual persona.

If you're a woman, find the row that corresponds with your sexual persona and then read the summary boxes for each of the male sexual personas, which are listed at the top of the page.

For men, you need to find the column that fits your sexual persona, and then read the boxes down the rows corresponding to the women's styles.

In each of the boxes, I listed the pros (ways your styles fit or complement each other) and the cons (ways your styles are different or potentially clash). Each box also has an up arrow (for a good fit), a down arrow (for a bad fit), or a sideways arrow (if it's unclear or could go either way).

In my studies, both men and women describe the power dynamic as the most pivotal factor shaping whether they click or not with a partner. If both of you want to be in charge or both of you expect the other person to take the lead, then sex tends to be stuck in first gear. Sex can be awkward or just go nowhere at all.

The overall level of sexual activity or intensity is ranked as the second most important factor. Most men and women want a partner who likes sex with the same level of movement and speed. If you really like sex that is slow and sensual, for example, you're going to be overwhelmed by a partner who likes fast, intense, and active sex.

The overall emotional tone of sex is also important, especially among men and women who prefer darker, sinful, and naughtier sex. When lovers from different sides of the emotional spectrum connect, the one with darker tastes will often be bored, and the one with more wholesome tastes will be intimidated or even scared!

As a rule of thumb, I gave pairings that matched on at least two out of three dimensions an up arrow, especially if their power dynamics complemented each other. Pairs that were mismatched on two out of three dimensions received a down arrow, especially if both personas had submissive styles or both liked to be in control.

Make a note of or circle the boxes with up arrows, since these are the sexual personas most likely to be compatible with your own. The odds are that one of these personas corresponds to the sexual persona you picked as ideal or most appealing in the previous section. If not, you're probably drawn to someone with a style that contrasts with your own. You may have a wholesome and innocent style, for example, but be drawn to a partner with a dark and naughty style.

Why Do Couples Click Despite Being Mismatched?

There's something overwhelming and discouraging about all the possible combinations in Exercise 4. Over the years, I've created lots of compatibility tables like this one to drive the matching algorithms for dating and relationship sites. There's something about mapping out every possible combination of fit that is both exhaustive and exhausting. When you think about all the possible ways that things can go wrong, it's a wonder any two people ever click sexually.

Plus, even if all the sexual style dimensions match up, there's still no guarantee that the two of you will have compatible sex drives or

Exercise 4: Likely Fit between Sexual Personas

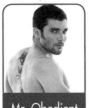
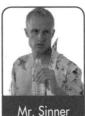
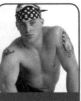
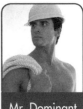

	Mr. Obedient	Mr. Sinner	Mr. Discipline	Mr. Dominant
Ms. Obedient 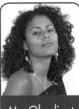	**PRO:** You share a dark and sensual approach to sex. **CON:** Both of you expect the other to take the lead sexually. **SUM:** ➲	**PRO:** You both like dark and sinful sex. **CON:** Neither of you like to take the lead. He likes it fast; she likes it slow. **SUM:** ☮	**PRO:** You both love naughty, sensual sex. He likes to take charge, and she loves to surrender. **CON:** None. **SUM:** ⋔	**PRO:** You're both drawn to dark, sinful sex. He enjoys taking control, and she enjoys surrendering. **CON:** He may be too rough for her. **SUM:** ⋔
Ms. Sinner 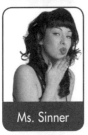	**PRO:** You both like dark and sinful sex. **CON:** Neither of you like to take the lead. She likes it fast; he likes it slow. **SUM:** ☮	**PRO:** You share a dark and intense approach to sex. **CON:** Both of you expect the other to take the lead sexually. **SUM:** ➲	**PRO:** You both like dark, sinful sex. She likes having a guy who takes charge. **CON:** He likes structure, while she's more uninhibited. **SUM:** ⋔	**PRO:** You both love wild, naughty, and uninhibited sex. He likes taking control, and she enjoys surrendering. **CON:** None. **SUM:** ⋔
Ms. Discipline 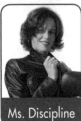	**PRO:** You both love naughty, sensual sex. She's strict and firm, and he enjoys having a woman take charge. **CON:** None. **SUM:** ⋔	**PRO:** You both like dark, sinful sex. He likes that she takes charge. **CON:** He tends to be uninhibited, while she is more strict and structured. **SUM:** ⋔	**PRO:** You share a dark and intense approach to sex. **CON:** Both of you like to be in control. You'll have to take turns being disciplined. **SUM:** ➲	**PRO:** You both like dark, sinful sex. **CON:** You both like to be in control. He may be too rough for her. **SUM:** ➲
Ms. Dominant 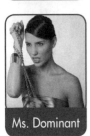	**PRO:** You're both drawn to dark, sinful sex. She enjoys taking control, and he enjoys surrendering. **CON:** He likes it slower; she likes it rougher. **SUM:** ⋔	**PRO:** You both love wild, naughty, and uninhibited sex. She likes taking control, and he enjoys surrendering. **CON:** None. **SUM:** ⋔	**PRO:** You both like dark, sinful sex. **CON:** You both like to be in control. Can you take turns? She may be too rough and intense for him. **SUM:** ➲	**PRO:** You both like wild, naughty, and uninhibited sex. **CON:** Both of you like to be in control. You'll have to take turns being on top. **SUM:** ➲

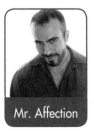 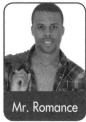 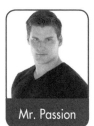 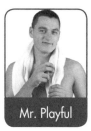

Mr. Affection	Mr. Romance	Mr. Passion	Mr. Playful

PRO: You both like it slow and sensual.

CON: He's wholesome; she's naughty. Both of you expect the other to take the lead sexually.

SUM: ☋

PRO: None.

CON: He'likes it wholesome and active; she likes it slow and naughty. Neither of you like to take the lead.

SUM: ☋

PRO: You're both sensual lovers. He likes to take charge, and she loves to surrender.

CON: She likes sex that's dark and sinful; he's more wholesome.

SUM: ☊

PRO: He likes to take charge, and she likes to surrender.

CON: She likes sex with a darker, more sensual tone. He likes it light and fast.

SUM: ➲

PRO: None.

CON: Neither of you like to take the lead. She likes it naughty and fast; he likes it wholesome and slow.

SUM: ☋

PRO: You both like sex that is fast and intense.

CON: She has a darker and more sinful approach to sex. Both of you expect the other to take the lead.

SUM: ☋

PRO: He likes to take charge; she likes to surrender.

CON: She likes wicked and intense sex. He likes it slow and wholesome.

SUM: ☋

PRO: You're both playful and intense lovers. He likes taking control, and she enjoys surrendering.

CON: Her sexual tastes are darker and naughtier.

SUM: ➲

PRO: You share a slow and sensual approach to sex. He enjoys having a woman who takes charge.

CON: She's likes sex with a darker and naughtier tone.

SUM: ☊

PRO: He likes that she takes charge.

CON: He has a light and uninhibited approach to sex, while she has a dark, sinful, and strict approach.

SUM: ➲

PRO: You both have a slow and sensual style.

CON: Both of you like to be in control. He likes sex when it's wholesome and kind; she likes it when it's sinful and dirty.

SUM: ☋

PRO: You both see sex as a powerful experience.

CON: You both like to be in control. He probably won't appreciate her dark and strict style.

SUM: ➲

PRO: You both enjoy slow, sensual sex. She enjoys taking control, and he enjoys surrendering.

CON: She likes darker and dirtier sex.

SUM: ☊

PRO: You both like active, uninhibited sex. She likes taking control, and he enjoys surrendering.

CON: She likes it dark and dirty; he's more wholesome.

SUM: ☊

PRO: None.

CON: You both like to be in control. She may be too rough and intense for him. He may be too innocent for her tastes.

SUM: ☋

PRO: You both like playful, uninhibited sex.

CON: Both of you like to be in control. She'll pull things in a dark and dirty direction; he'll try to keep it light and fun.

SUM: ☋

Instructions

Women: Find the row with your <u>Sexual Persona</u>. Read the summary of fits with the eight male personas listed in columns.

Men: Find the column with your <u>Sexual Persona</u>. Read the summary of fits with the eight female personas listed in rows.

KEY:

☊ Good Fit

➲ Mediocre

☋ Poor Fit

Exercise 4 (continued)

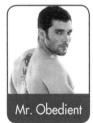

Mr. Obedient

Mr. Sinner

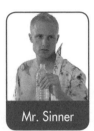

Mr. Discipline

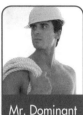

Mr. Dominant

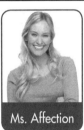

Ms. Affection

PRO: You share a slow and sensual approach to sex.

CON: Both of you expect the other to take the lead sexually. He likes it dark and dirty; she's more wholesome.

SUM: ☽

PRO: None

CON: Neither of you like to take the lead. He likes it fast; she likes it slow. He likes it sinful; she likes it wholesome.

SUM: ☽

PRO: You're both very sensual lovers. He likes to take charge, and she loves to surrender.

CON: His sexual interests are darker and naughtier than hers.

SUM: ♈

PRO: He enjoys taking control, and she enjoys surrendering.

CON: He may be too rough for her. She may be too wholesome and innocent for him.

SUM: ⊃

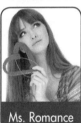

Ms. Romance

PRO: None

CON: Neither of you like to take the lead. She likes sex sinful and fast; he likes it wholesome and slow.

SUM: ☽

PRO: You both enjoy active and very physical sex.

CON: Both of you expect the other to take the lead sexually. His sexual tastes are darker than hers.

SUM: ⊃

PRO: She likes having a guy who takes charge.

CON: He likes discipline and structure, while she's more wholesome and uninhibited.

SUM: ⊃

PRO: You both love wild and uninhibited sex. He likes taking control, and she enjoys surrendering.

CON: His sexual tastes are darker than hers.

SUM: ♈

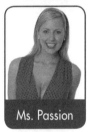

Ms. Passion

PRO: You both like slow and sensual sex. He likes strong women who take charge.

CON: He likes dark and naughty sex; she's more wholesome.

SUM: ♈

PRO: He likes that she takes charge.

CON: He likes sinful, naughty, and uninhibited sex. She likes it slow, sensual, and wholesome.

SUM: ⊃

PRO: You share a slow and intense approach to sex.

CON: Both of you like to be in control. He'll pull sex in a darker and naughtier direction than she likes.

SUM: ☽

PRO: None.

CON: You both like to be in control. He'll pull sex in a dark and wild direction; she'll want to keep things sensual and wholesome.

SUM: ☽

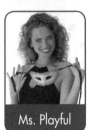

Ms. Playful

PRO: She enjoys taking the lead; he likes to surrender.

CON: He likes it slow she likes it fast. He likes sex on the darker side; she's more wholesome.

SUM: ⊃

PRO: You both enjoy active and very physical sex. She likes taking control, and he likes to surrender.

CON: His sexual tastes are darker than hers.

SUM: ♈

PRO: You share a slow and sensual approach to sex.

CON: You both like to be in control. He'll pull sex in a darker and naughtier direction than she likes.

SUM: ⊃

PRO: You both like active and uninhibited sex.

CON: Both of you like to be in control. He'll pull sex in a dark and sinful direction; she's more wholesome.

SUM: ⊃

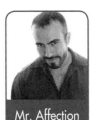 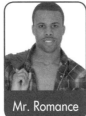 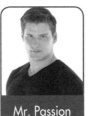 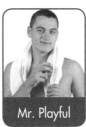

| Mr. Affection | Mr. Romance | Mr. Passion | Mr. Playful |

PRO: You both like slow , sensual, and wholesome sex.

CON: Both of you expect the other to take the lead sexually.

SUM: ➲

PRO: You share a wholesome approach to sex.

CON: He likes active and physical sex; she likes it slow and sensual. Neither of you like to take the lead.

SUM: ☹

PRO: You share a slow, sensual, and wholesome sexual style. He likes to take charge, and she loves to surrender.

CON: None

SUM: ☺

PRO: You share a wholesome approach to sex. He likes to take charge, and she likes to surrender.

CON: He likes it fast; she likes it slow and sensual.

SUM: ➲

PRO: You share a wholesome approach to sex.

CON: Neither of you like to take the lead. She likes it fast; he likes it slow and sensual.

SUM: ☹

PRO: You share a fun, active , and wholesome approach to sex.

CON: Both of you expect the other to take the lead.

SUM: ➲

PRO: You share an innocent and wholesome style. He likes to take charge; she likes to surrender.

CON: She likes it fast; he likes it slow and sensual.

SUM: ➲

PRO: You're both playful, active, and intense lovers. He likes taking control, and she enjoys surrendering.

CON: None

SUM: ☺

PRO: You share a slow , sensual, and wholesome approach to sex. He enjoys having a woman who takes charge.

CON: None

SUM: ☺

PRO: You share an innocent and wholesome approach to sex. He likes that she takes charge.

CON: She likes it fast; he likes it slow.

SUM: ☺

PRO: You both have a slow, sensual, and wholesome style.

CON: Both of you like to be in control. Can you take turns being on top?

SUM: ➲

PRO: You share a wholesome and fun approach to sex.

CON: You both like to be in control. He likes it fast and active; she likes it slow and sensual.

SUM: ☹

PRO: You share a wholesome approach to sex. She enjoys taking control; he enjoys surrendering.

CON: She likes it fast; he likes it slow.

SUM: ☺

PRO: You both like active, fun, and uninhibited sex. She likes taking control; he enjoys surrendering.

CON: None

SUM: ☺

PRO: You share a wholesome approach to sex.

CON: You both like to be in control. She likes it fast; he likes it slow and sensual.

SUM: ☹

PRO: You both like playful, fun, and uninhibited sex.

CON: Both of you like to be in control. Can you take turns being on top?

SUM: ➲

KEY:

☺ Good Fit

➲ Mediocre

☹ Poor Fit

be into the same sexual activities. As you'll see in the next section, it's hard to predict your compatibility in sex drive or sexual adventurousness even if you know a lover's sexual persona.

Yet obviously lots of couples hit it off, even when their sexual styles are mismatched on one or all the dimensions. Why is that?

The importance of these matches (or mismatches) depends in part on how strong your preference is on each of the dimensions. Remember that the preferences for emotional tone, power, and activity vary on a continuum. Some people have strong and firm preferences on either end of the continuum, but most of us fall somewhere in between and have some flexibility in what we enjoy or what we need in order to be turned on sexually.

If you *only* enjoy sex that is dark, sinful, and naughty and connect with someone who *only* likes sex that is wholesome, pure, and innocent, then emotional tone is probably going to be a deal breaker. But most men and women can find some compromise in styles that makes sex "naughty enough" but still "wholesome enough" to satisfy both of their preferences.

The same goes for fits on the activity dimension. If you like it fast, and your partner likes it slow, you can probably slow things down and be sensual, especially if you see how much this turns him or her on. Then you can get fast and intense when you get close to your climax. Most couples find ways to divide their sexual time so that each person gets to enjoy sex in their favorite zone for at least part of the time.

Matches on the power dimension can be trickier. There are some combinations that clearly do not work. If you have a strong preference for being dominant or being submissive, then you will probably be frustrated (and maybe even turned off) by a partner who can't give you what you need. People who fit into these extreme power dynamics tend to have kinkier sexual tastes. As we'll see in the next section, having Kinky tastes adds an additional layer of complexity to matching.

However, for most men and women with Vanilla or Mainstream sexual tastes, preferences for power dynamics tend to be somewhat flexible. If both partners have gentle or passive styles, the two may take turns initiating and taking charge during sex. If both partners are more forceful and dominant, they can take turns being on top or being in control.

If given the option, compatibility is certainly easier when you find a partner with a matching sexual persona. In Part 4 we'll look at ways to find and attract a partner with a style that fits with your own. Still, ending up in a relationship with mismatched styles is not the end of the world. In Chapter 12 we'll look at ways to satisfy both of your sexual styles and create a more compatible connection.

Is HOW You Approach Sex Linked to WHAT You Like to Do Sexually?

Ideally, you want to find a find a partner with a style that matches yours *and* who enjoys the same amount and variety of sex. In Chapter 3 we looked at whether external personality traits predicted sexual interests. We learned that there was an imperfect connection between public personas and sex drive and adventurousness. You can't always judge a book by its cover, but there are definitely trends where you can expect certain public personas (like Adventurer or Rebel) to want sex more often and with a more adventurous flair than people with other personas (like Shy or Nice).

Now we can look specifically at personality as it relates to our sexual selves and explore whether the sexual personas predict sexual interests. In other words, does *how* you approach sex relate to how often you want sex and *what* you like to do sexually?

My research suggests there is a pretty strong (although still imperfect) link between the sexual personas and sex drive and adventurousness. I've summarized the findings in Figure 3 (for women) and Figure 4 (for men). For each sexual persona, the figures list the percentage of women or men with *high* or *very high* sex drives and the percentage with Adventurous or Kinky sexual tastes.

Figure 3: Sex Drive and Adventurousness of Women's Sexual Personas

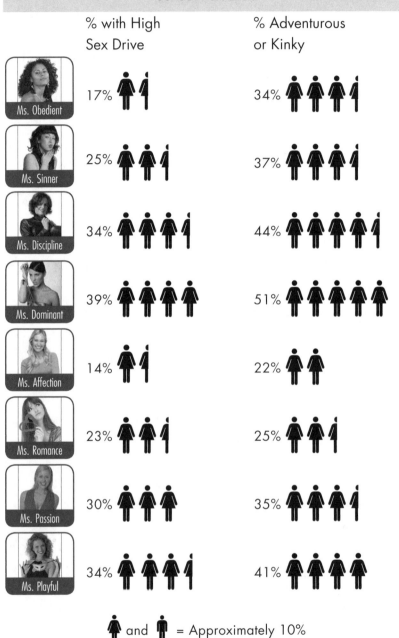

	% with High Sex Drive	% Adventurous or Kinky
Ms. Obedient	17%	34%
Ms. Sinner	25%	37%
Ms. Discipline	34%	44%
Ms. Dominant	39%	51%
Ms. Affection	14%	22%
Ms. Romance	23%	25%
Ms. Passion	30%	35%
Ms. Playful	34%	41%

👤 and 👤 = Approximately 10%

Figure 4: Sex Drive and Adventurousness of Men's Sexual Personas

	% with High Sex Drive	% Adventurous or Kinky
Mr. Obedient	23%	43%
Mr. Sinner	30%	48%
Mr. Discipline	39%	54%
Mr. Dominant	45%	60%
Mr. Affection	19%	25%
Mr. Romance	25%	31%
Mr. Passion	38%	40%
Mr. Playful	42%	44%

and = Approximately 10%

Who Is the Most (and Least) Likely to Want Lots and Lots of Kinky Sex?

Let's start by pointing out the sexual personas who are the most likely to have high sex drives and high adventurousness. Among both men and women, four personas stand out. These are the four styles with dominant power: Discipline, Dominant, Passion, and Playful.

Combining dominance with negative emotional tone and/or a fast style also appears to increase the likelihood of wanting more sex and more adventurous sex. In fact, men and women with the Mr. or Ms. Dominant style that combines these factors are the most likely to have high sexual desire and high adventurousness. So being strong, forceful, bold, and uninhibited in bed often goes hand in hand with wanting a lot of sex and wanting to test sexual limits and to explore a variety of sexual activities and positions.

Lower sexual desire and less adventurousness are associated with sexual personas with a positive emotional tone, low power, and slow activity. In fact, Mr. or Ms. Affection, which combines these factors, is the persona most likely to have a low sexual drive and Mainstream sexual tastes. Having a partner with a warm, sensual, and tender sexual style can be wonderful as long as you don't expect or need to have sex every day or want to try out lots of new sexual activities or positions.

Obviously, these are trends, not absolutes. You'll recall from Part 1 that most men and women have low or moderate sex drives and have Vanilla or Mainstream sexual tastes. So, not surprisingly, the majority of men and women across all the sexual personas have low or moderate sex drives. In other words, regardless of which sexual persona you meet in the bedroom, chances are he or she will *not* want sex every day or have a crazy high sex drive.

If that's what you're looking for in a partner, your best chance is with either Mr. or Ms. Dominant or Mr. or Ms. Playful. If you meet a woman with one of these two personas, there's a one in three chance that she'll have a high sex drive. If you meet a man with a

Dominant or Playful style, there's a fifty-fifty chance that he'll want sex every day.

It's a little easier to predict sexual adventurousness than it is to predict sex drive. Among men, two personas stand out as being especially likely to be Adventurous or Kinky. If you connect with Mr. Discipline or Mr. Dominant, your chances are greater than 50 percent that he will like a lot of sexual variety and prefer wilder, naughtier, or kinkier sex. The same is true with one of the women's personas. Over half of the women who fit in the Ms. Dominant category prefer Adventurous or Kinky sex. Of course, half of them do not. So it's certainly possible to have a Dominant style and still prefer sexual activities that are relatively tame or only moderately adventurous.

PART 4

Improving Your Sexual Chemistry

Chapter 11

Finding a Sexual Persona That Fits Yours

Sex and Dating

What Is the Biggest Challenge in Finding a Compatible Partner?

Now that we've looked at the multiple ingredients that go into creating sexual chemistry, let's look at several strategies for finding a partner with a sexual persona that meshes with your own. If you're already in a relationship, you may want to skip to Chapter 12, where we look at ways to sustain and enhance your sexual chemistry.

Finding a partner whom you connect with on multiple sexual levels isn't easy. In Part 2 we looked at some of the challenges single folks face in trying to find a partner with a similar sex drive and similar sexual interests. Ideally, these are issues couples should talk about before they get too deep into a relationship. Compared to sexual chemistry, issues of sex drives and sexual adventurousness are relatively straightforward. You can learn through experience how often your partner likes to have sex and discover over time how much sexual variety he or she wants or needs.

Sexual chemistry is a more mysterious and elusive phenomenon. When it's there, you know it. But when it's missing, it can be hard to put your finger on what's not working. This is especially baffling if you're really attracted to the person you're dating or have started to fall in love with each other. When you have a great emotional connection with someone outside the bedroom, you expect this will naturally carry over into your sexual connection.

However, if your sexual personas do not mesh, you are both going to be frustrated. You're both going to want things emotionally and sexually that your partner is not going to feel comfortable giving. As we'll see in the next chapter, I believe there are things couples can do to understand and meet each other's needs and realign their sexual connection. It's not impossible to overcome mismatched sexual personas, but it's not easy either. That's why it's important to seek out potential partners who share the basic ingredients of good sexual chemistry.

In this chapter we're going to revisit the types of sexual qualities you find exciting and sexy. We'll look at how the range of qualities you're drawn to shapes the size of your dating pool. We'll also look at the advantages and disadvantages of having versatile sexual tastes. If you enjoy playing multiple different sexual roles, you probably need to find a partner who also has a versatile sexual style.

We'll look at how most men and women try to judge a book by its cover and guess a potential date's sexual style based on his or her body type or looks. Although these assumptions and expectations are very common, they do not tend to be very accurate. Instead, I'll show you how to watch for clues in people's behavior and their public personality that can help you to predict their sexual style.

Finally, I'll offer a few words of advice on embracing sexual complexity in yourself and your potential partners. We'll look at several things you can do to highlight your sexual personality and to communicate with dates and potential partners about your sexual side.

What Is the Range of Qualities That Turns You On?

In Chapter 10 we focused on identifying a single sexual persona that you found especially appealing. But now that we're looking at your dating life and all the potential people you can date, it makes sense to expand our scope and look at *all* the sexual personas you find appealing.

To do this, let's take a second look at the qualities you find attractive in a lover. Take a moment to complete Exercises 1 and 2. Start on the left side of the page and circle all the qualities you find especially sexy in a lover. Then, on the right side of the page, circle the terms that describe your own personal sexual style.

I realize some of these terms could apply to your public personality and how you think and act in nonsexual contexts. However, for the purpose of these exercises, try to focus on how these qualities apply to your sex life, what you're looking for in a lover, and what you bring to your partner as a lover.

When I was a teenager, my friends and I used to read fortune cookies by adding the phrase "in bed" to the end of the fortune. For example, "You are popular and loved by your friends...in bed," "You will find success in a new business venture...in bed," and so forth. So try taking the same approach with the terms in these exercises.

In Exercise 1, on the left side of the page, ask yourself if you are attracted to a partner who is

- bold...in bed?
- goofy...in bed?
- intense...in bed?
- bashful...in bed?

Then in Exercise 2, on the right side of the page, circle all of the qualities *you* embody sexually. Which traits do you take on when you're having sex? How would you describe yourself in bed?

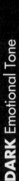

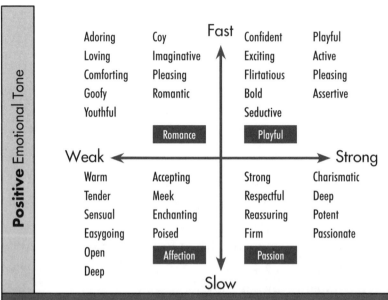

Positive Emotional Tone

Fast

Adoring	Coy	Confident	Playful
Loving	Imaginative	Exciting	Active
Comforting	Pleasing	Flirtatious	Pleasing
Goofy	Romantic	Bold	Assertive
Youthful		Seductive	

Romance   Playful

Weak ←————————————————→ Strong

Warm	Accepting	Strong	Charismatic
Tender	Meek	Respectful	Deep
Sensual	Enchanting	Reassuring	Potent
Easygoing	Poised	Firm	Passionate
Open	Affection	Passion	
Deep			

Slow

Exercise 1: Circle the traits you find especially sexy in a lover.

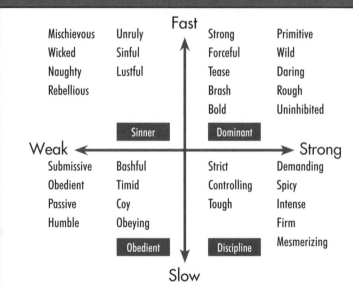

DARK Emotional Tone

Fast

Mischievous	Unruly	Strong	Primitive
Wicked	Sinful	Forceful	Wild
Naughty	Lustful	Tease	Daring
Rebellious		Brash	Rough
		Bold	Uninhibited

Sinner   Dominant

Weak ←————————————————→ Strong

Submissive	Bashful	Strict	Demanding
Obedient	Timid	Controlling	Spicy
Passive	Coy	Tough	Intense
Humble	Obeying		Firm
	Obedient	Discipline	Mesmerizing

Slow

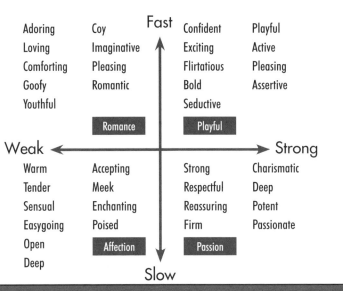

Exercise 2: Circle your sexual traits.

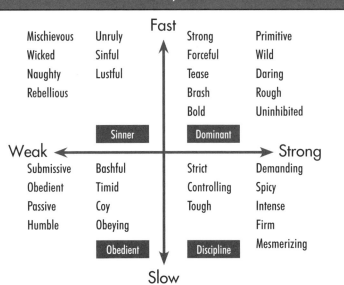

After you are done with both exercises, the terms you circled will probably look like a cloud or several clouds. Take a look at the left side of the page. If the cloud of circled terms is focused in a single quadrant, then you have a clear preference for a single sexual persona.

If the cloud of circled terms goes across quadrants or there are multiple clouds, then you are attracted to multiple sexual personas. There are two ways of looking at this. Let's consider the best-case scenario first.

How Big Is Your Potential Dating Pool?

People who are open to dating multiple sexual personas dramatically increase their potential dating pool. I have listed the proportion of men and women who fit in each of the sexual persona categories in Exercise 3. Put a check beside each of the sexual personas you find attractive or consider compatible with your own. Then add up the percentages associated with each. This sum is the potential size of your dating pool *if* you are open to a partner with any of your favorite sexual personas.

Another way to approach this is to put an X through sexual personas that you are definitely *not* attracted to. Identify any of the types that you believe would be incompatible with your own. Add up the percentages associated with the sexual personas you have ruled out. At a minimum, you can reduce the scope of your dating pool by this amount.

Obviously, the larger your potential dating pool, the better your odds of finding a partner whom you will find sexy in bed. Since there are no perfect predictors of sexual personas based on either appearance or personality, there is always a potential for a bedroom surprise. But the larger the sum in Exercise 3, the better your odds of liking the person your lover becomes when the clothes come off.

The other possibility is that you want a partner who can embody *all* of the qualities you circled. This is a more challenging scenario,

Exercise 3: Sum the Proportion You Find Attractive

	Check the Sexual Personas You Find Attractive		Check the Sexual Personas You Find Attractive
Ms. Obedient	☐ 9%	Mr. Obedient	☐ 10%
Ms. Sinner	☐ 14%	Mr. Sinner	☐ 12%
Ms. Discipline	☐ 6%	Mr. Discipline	☐ 7%
Ms. Dominant	☐ 8%	Mr. Dominant	☐ 8%
Ms. Affection	☐ 16%	Mr. Affection	☐ 17%
Ms. Romance	☐ 23%	Mr. Romance	☐ 17%
Ms. Passion	☐ 10%	Mr. Passion	☐ 13%
Ms. Playful	☐ 14%	Mr. Playful	☐ 16%
Sum the Percentage of Personas You Find Attractive:	○		○

because rather than increasing the size of your dating pool, you have added more restrictions. Now, not only does your lover need to fit one sexual persona, he or she also needs to be versatile enough to embody other roles as well.

There is nothing wrong with wanting it all. You simply have to be aware of your odds and be willing to do some extra work to find a compatible partner. More on that in a moment, but first let's take a look at how wide or narrow your own sexual personality tends to be.

What Are the Advantages and Disadvantages of Being Versatile?

Go back and look at Exercise 2 and the terms you circled to describe your own sexual style. If the cloud of circled terms is isolated in a single quadrant, then you have a single sexual persona. If there are multiple clouds of circled terms that describe you, then you can embody multiple sexual personas. Back in Chapter 7 you probably fit into one of the *versatile* power categories. You probably enjoy taking the lead sexually sometimes, but you also enjoy surrendering control at other times. You may have discovered in previous chapters that you enjoy both the light and darker sides of sexuality. You may enjoy fast and intense play as well as slow and sensual play.

At first glance, you might expect a versatile person would have more sexual options. This is partially true. Being able to embody multiple sexual personas certainly increases the odds of fitting into what a new lover might be looking for. Looking for a Mr. Romance? No problem, I can be that. Looking for Mr. Dominant? I can be that too!

However, when it comes to *relationships*, versatile men and women can be more difficult to match, not less. That's because versatile individuals usually don't want to stay in a single sexual role. They enjoy switching between roles. They may want to play a dominant role one evening, then be submissive the next. They may be sweet and tender one night, then wild and rough the next. Some versatile folks like to cover all this territory in a single evening.

Not everyone can keep up with a versatile man or woman. The ideal match is an equally versatile person who enjoys being versatile in the same way. If this describes you, then it's important to appreciate that you're special and have special needs. You're going to have to do a lot of searching to find a partner who shares your versatile interests.

Predicting Sexual Personas

Do You Make Assumptions about People's Sexual Interests Based on Their Looks?

I wish there were an easy way to tell what a person's sexual persona is likely to be ahead of time. If you have a casual attitude toward sex, then you probably don't mind trying out new lovers and learning through trial and error who fits and who doesn't. However, for those of us with less casual attitudes, the process of dating, forming emotional attachments, and then testing out your sexual chemistry with potential new partners can be frustrating and exhausting.

So it's understandable that many men and women do their best to short-cut this frustration and try to anticipate ahead of time the type of lover a person is likely to be. Most of their assumptions seem to focus on physical qualities like body type and facial features, but people also tend to read a lot into clothing and hairstyles.

A few years ago I decided to do a study where I asked people to guess what type of lover a person would be simply based on a photo of that person. I was worried that most of the subjects would either refuse to guess or answer "unsure" for most of the questions. After all, these were detailed and explicit questions: Is she a passionate lover? Does he prefer mild or wild sex? Is he more dominant or submissive sexually? And so forth.

Much to my surprise, not only did everyone *have* an opinion about the sexual proclivities of the people in the photos, but they gave their answers in record time. They made their judgments quickly, and most said they expected their guesses were extremely accurate.

I used some of the photos from these studies to illustrate the different sexual styles in the previous chapters. I picked photos that tended to remind people of certain sexual qualities. A man in a black T-shirt with tattoos on his arms, for example, fits what most people think of when they imagine a sexual Rebel. A smiling woman in a pretty dress looks like she would be a Romantic.

Advertisers and movie producers associate physical types with certain personality types all the time. In a two-hour movie, we don't have time to get to know the background and complexities of every character. The plot can move more quickly if the hero looks like a hero, victims look like victims, villains look like villains, and so forth. So we've all been inundated with these assumptions from thousands of hours of television, hundreds of movies, and millions of advertisements.

Take a moment to check out either Exercise 4 (for women) or Exercise 5 (for men) and see whether you associate certain sexual qualities with these photographs. What kind of lover would you expect each person to be? After you've made your ratings, you can see how most other men and women rated the photos. If your ratings were similar, then your assumptions are in line with most other men and women. If not, then you either make fewer assumptions about sexual personality or you have your own unique set of assumptions.

In my studies, the most consistent assumptions people make based on appearances center on issues of emotional tone and power. Most of these assumptions fit what I would describe as gender stereotypes.

Women who look mature, have serious facial expressions, or have prominent facial features (like a larger nose or a strong chin) are assumed to be powerful and assertive lovers. They're also assumed to like sex with darker and more sinful tones.

In contrast, women who look girlish (regardless of their chronological age) have soft smiles or delicate facial features and are assumed to be sexually passive and innocent. Most men also tend to assume that these girlish-looking women prefer sex that is loving, gentle, and affectionate.

Men are not the only ones who make assumptions about sexual interests based on looks. Most women believe you can tell something about a man's sexual style based on his body type and facial features.

Men who are big and muscular and look tough and serious in their photos are assumed to be dominant and aggressive lovers and prefer sex with a darker emotional tone. In contrast, men with big smiles, boyish looks, or more feminine features are assumed to be gentle, tender, and sensual lovers.

Are Expectations Based on Looks Usually Accurate?

While it's clear from my studies that lots of men and women make these sorts of assumptions, I've found no evidence that these predictions tend to be true.

You find the same wide variety of sexual interests among girlish-looking women as you do among more mature or masculine-looking women. Muscular or big men are no more likely to be assertive or dominant lovers than boyish-looking or thin men.

Life would be a lot easier if you could judge a book by its cover. But so far I've found no connection between how people look and their sexual persona.

Where Can I Find the Best Clues into a Potential Partner's Sexual Style?

The best clues to watch for if you're trying to guess someone's sexual persona probably come from their behavior and personality

Exercise 4: Judging Women's Sexual Persona

	What Do You Expect Her Sexual Style Would Be? (Circle Your Choice)	What Most Men Expected
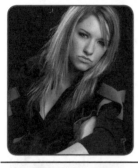	**Dark** *or* **Positive** **Gentle** *or* **Powerful** **Slow** *or* **Fast**	*Dark* *Powerful* *Fast*
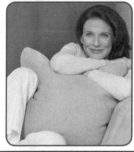	**Dark** *or* **Positive** **Gentle** *or* **Powerful** **Slow** *or* **Fast**	*Positive* *Gentle* *Slow*
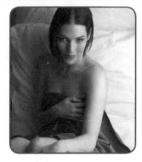	**Dark** *or* **Positive** **Gentle** *or* **Powerful** **Slow** *or* **Fast**	*Dark* *Gentle* *Slow*

Exercise 5: Judging Men's Sexual Persona

	What Do You Expect His Sexual Style Would Be? (Circle Your Choice)	What Most Women Expected
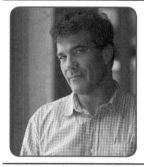	**Dark** *or* **Positive** **Gentle** *or* **Powerful** **Slow** *or* **Fast**	*Positive* *Powerful* *Slow*
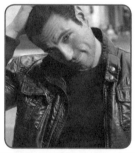	**Dark** *or* **Positive** **Gentle** *or* **Powerful** **Slow** *or* **Fast**	*Dark* *Powerful* *Fast*
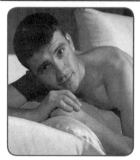	**Dark** *or* **Positive** **Gentle** *or* **Powerful** **Slow** *or* **Fast**	*Positive* *Gentle* *Slow*

rather than their looks. As I mentioned in the last chapter, public personalities and sexual personalities are two distinct things and can exist in a variety of combinations. Still, some combinations appear to be more common than others. In my studies I've found a consistent link between several of the public personas and some of the sexual personas.

Once you know a date's public persona, you can usually *narrow down* the set of sexual personas that he or she is likely to have. So even though you can't be 100 percent sure about someone's sexual style based on their external traits, there are definitely a few clues to watch for that can point you in the right direction.

In Figure 1 I've listed for each of the public personas the three or four most common sexual personas for that type. You may want to flip back to Chapter 3 and remind yourself of the public personas you find most appealing. Then take a look at Figure 1 and see if the sexual persona you're drawn to is listed beside your favorite public persona. If so, then your chances of encountering surprises in the bedroom are reduced, because the type of external personality you find attractive tends to concur with a sexual style you find appealing.

If your favorite sexual persona is *not* listed beside your favorite public persona, it does not mean that the two never go together. It's simply a rare combination. So your chances of a bedroom surprise go up.

Can I Predict Whether They Like the Lighter or Darker Side of Sex?

The connection between public personality and sexual chemistry is strongest on two of the three sexual dimensions: emotional tone and activity. Let's start by looking at some of the personality clues to watch for, depending on whether you're drawn to the lighter or darker side of sex.

Figure 1: Common Sexual Personas for Each Public Persona

Public Personas	Most Common Sexual Personas

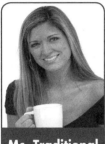 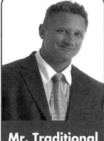

Ms. Traditional **Mr. Traditional**

 Ms. Affection   Ms. Romance

 Mr. Obedient  Mr. Discipline   Mr. Affection   Mr. Romance

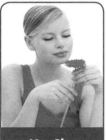 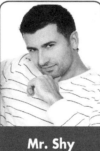

Ms. Shy **Mr. Shy**

 Ms. Obedient   Ms. Sinner   Ms. Affection Ms. Romance

 Mr. Obedient   Mr. Sinner   Mr. Affection   Mr. Romance

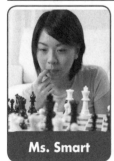 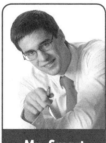

Ms. Smart **Mr. Smart**

 Ms. Obedient   Ms. Sinner   Ms. Dominant

 Mr. Obedient Mr. Sinner Mr. Dominant   Mr. Playful

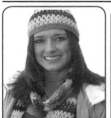 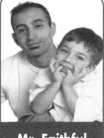

Ms. Faithful **Mr. Faithful**

 Ms. Sinner   Ms. Affection Ms. Romance Ms. Playful

 Mr. Sinner Mr. Affection   Mr. Romance  Mr. Playful

Figure 1 (continued)

Public Personas		Most Common Sexual Personas

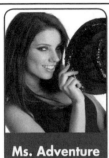 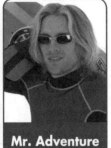

 Ms. Dominant Ms. Romance Ms. Passion Ms. Playful

 Mr. Dominant Mr. Affection Mr. Romance Mr. Passion

Ms. Adventure **Mr. Adventure**

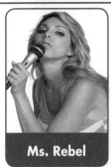 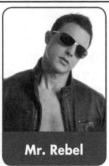

 Ms. Sinner Ms. Dominant Ms. Playful

 Mr. Sinner Mr. Dominant Mr. Passion Mr. Playful

Ms. Rebel **Mr. Rebel**

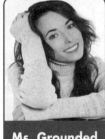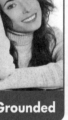 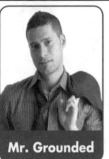

 Ms. Sinner Ms. Affection Ms. Romance

Mr. Affection Mr. Romance Mr. Passion Mr. Playful

 Ms. Grounded **Mr. Grounded**

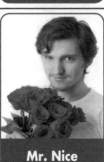

 Ms. Affection 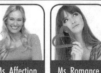 Ms. Romance Ms. Passion Ms. Playful

 Mr. Affection Mr. Romance Mr. Passion Mr. Playful

Ms. Nice **Mr. Nice**

As you can see in Figure 1, the most common sexual personas associated with the Smart personality type are linked to the darker side of sex. In fact, if you meet Mr. or Ms. Smart, the chances are greater than 50 percent that this individual will have a sexual persona with a dark emotional tone. So if you're looking for a partner who is wicked, naughty, or wild in bed, keep an eye out for individuals with a public side that is creative, talented, and original.

In contrast, if you meet someone with the Grounded personality type, this individual will almost certainly have a sexual persona with a positive emotional tone. This is the case among both men and women, but it especially applies to women. In fact, over half of the Ms. Grounded women fall in either the Ms. Affection or Ms. Romance categories. So if you meet someone whose public personality is trusting, practical, and relaxed, then chances are good that he or she is going to approach sex in a tender, warm, and affectionate way. In other words, if the person you're dating is modest and down-to-earth, he or she is probably not going to be wild and nasty sexually.

We see the same consistency between the public and private side of personality among people with the Nice persona. About two out of three men and women with the Nice persona prefer sex that has a light or fun emotional tone. So only rarely will you find someone who is warm, friendly, and kind on the outside who has a private sexual side that is primitive, dark, and nasty. So if you like nice guys (or gals), I hope you also like tender and wholesome sex.

Can I Predict If They Have a Fast or Slow Sexual Style?

I've heard several interesting folk theories about how to predict the type of lover someone is going to be. Dating expert Tracey Cox, for example, recommends paying attention to how your date eats.[43] She believes that dates who woof down their meal tend to be the "wham, bam, thank-you, ma'am" type, while dates who savor each morsel tend to be slow and patient lovers who would take their time enjoying your body.

I have a friend who swears you can tell the kind of lover someone will be by how he or she dances. According to him, a woman who just stands and sways while she dances will expect you to do all the work sexually, while a bouncy, energetic dancer will be bouncy and exciting in bed.

I even have my own folk theory about predicting a lover's sexual pace. I love to hike and often take friends (and occasionally a date) along with me. Based on my experience, there are two kinds of hikers, and this tends to correspond with two sexual styles. The first type focuses on the destination, hikes at a brisk pace, and does a lot of bragging and high-fiving when we reach the peak. The second type enjoys a slower pace, lingers by streams, stops and smells the flowers, and soaks in the views. Both can be fun experiences. It just depends on the mood you're in.[44] When I hike on my own, I have my own preferred pace, but I won't go into that, since it would be too revealing.

Aside from these unscientific theories, what does the research tell us about who tends to have slow or fast sexual styles? As you can see in Figure 1, the strongest link between public personality and sexual style on the activity dimension exists for the Shy persona. If you meet either Mr. or Ms. Shy, this individual will almost certainly have a sexual persona that approaches sex with slow intensity (such as Mr. or Ms. Obedient, Sinner, Affection, or Romance). So Shy individuals who tend to be gentle, mild mannered, and reserved in their public life tend to approach sex in a similar slow and deliberate way.

How Are Traditional Men Tricky?

It turns out that a Traditional public personality offers fairly good clues about sexual interests among women but not among men. The vast majority of Traditional women fall in either the Ms. Affection or Ms. Romance categories. So if you meet a woman who is confident, conservative, and hard-working, you can pretty much count on the fact that she will prefer sex that is light and positive and prefer to play a more passive and submissive role sexually. It is rare to find a Traditional woman with a hidden sexual side that is dark, wild, or dominant.

Traditional men, though, are all over the map sexually. I listed the four most common sexual personas for this type in Figure 1, but in fact, Traditional men are represented across all eight of the sexual personas.

This makes dates with Traditional men especially prone to bedroom surprises. You can expect Mr. Traditional to act confident, assertive, and conservative on your date. But when the lights go down and the clothes come off, he is equally likely to be a kinky Mr. Obedient as he is a mild-manner Mr. Romance.

Opening Up about Your Sexual Side

How Can You Describe Your Sexual Style?

As we've seen throughout this book, sexuality is a complex and multifaceted phenomenon. Although there are some interesting connections between public personas and sexual personas, consistency between our public selves and our private selves seems to be the exception rather than the rule.

My advice is to embrace this complexity. Embrace it in yourself. Don't force your sexuality into a neat box that fits your external personality. Don't waste your time trying to be the person people expect you to be, based on your looks.

Most of us spend our lives reacting to how other people see us. We react to their expectations and assumptions about who we are and what we like.

To break out of this trap, you need a proactive plan for how you're going to communicate with dates and potential partners about your sexual side. Just like big companies develop communication plans to sell you on the benefits and advantages of their products, you need a plan that highlights your best features and shows the real you in all your rich complexity.

Let's start by picking a set of words you can use to describe your sexual persona. Flip back and take a look at the words you circled to describe yourself in Exercise 2. I want you to think about how you can use these terms to describe yourself in a general way and then in a more explicit sexual way.

Developing a vocabulary to describe your sexual side can be helpful whether you're dating online or off-line. But the terms can be especially useful online. For example, you can use these terms to create a rich and compelling personal profile on dating websites or social networking sites (like Facebook or MySpace).

First, you need to pick several descriptive terms that are not explicitly sexual. Terms like *playful, loving, active,* and *goofy* fit into this category. You can use these adjectives to describe your general personality, but they also make it easy to imagine the type of lover you would be.

On the next level are terms that have a sexual meaning but are still general enough that you can use them without explicitly referencing sex. When you use words like *tender, passionate, flirtatious, daring,* or *uninhibited* to describe yourself, you can point to your sexual side without spelling it out.

Advertisers do this all the time. They link cars, shampoos, and even breakfast cereals with sexual imagery and use words like *bold, daring,* and *exciting* to make implicit associations between their products and sex. You can do the same thing by painting a picture of yourself with these subtly sexual words.

In my research one of the things that set successful online daters apart from those who fail to find a relationship online is their ability to communicate in a sexy and engaging way. They are able to paint themselves as passionate and sexual people without being overly explicit or scaring potential dates off by being too forward or gross.

Personally, I don't see anything wrong in describing both your public personality and your sexual side as part of your profile, as long as you use some restraint and subtlety. If you have a high sex drive, it makes sense to talk about the type of sexual connection you're looking for. In which case, you can use phrases like *high sex drive*, *sexually adventurous*, or *kinky* and describe the type of sex you enjoy. If you enjoy taking charge sexually, say so. If you enjoy sex that is wild and naughty, spell it out. To be honest, this will probably scare away more conservative types and people with low sex drives, but if you have a high sex drive, it's good to weed these folks out from the start.

What If Your Sexual Self Is Very Different from Your Public Personality?

I believe everyone can benefit from having a personal communication plan. But this is especially important if your sexual persona is different from your public personality. The bigger the gap is between your public self and private sexuality, the greater the risk that potential dates will have inaccurate expectations about what you like sexually. You also risk missing potentially great sexual connections, because potential dates don't see in your external features the qualities they are looking for in a lover. So you have to learn how to advertise all the great stuff you have to offer sexually that is hidden from view.

Your online profile can be a great place to paint a picture of your public side and your private side. You can do this with descriptive terms like the ones in Exercises 1 and 2 as well as photographs that show how you embody these qualities.

Take a look at each of the photographs on your profile page and ask yourself: What emotional tone does this convey? Does it show me as light, fun, and pleasant or dark, naughty, and mysterious? If your public persona is Mr. Nice, but your sexual persona is Mr. Sinner, you want to include words *and* images in your profile that show you can embody both ends of the emotional continuum. It's great to include photos of you laughing and having fun with your friends, but you also need a couple of photos that show your rebellious and dark side. If you have a photo of you on a motorcycle with a leather jacket and looking tough, now's the time to pull it out!

As we saw earlier, most men and women make assumptions about people's sexual personas based on their appearances. So it makes sense to look the part in your online profile and when you go on dates.

Of course, your online profile can't communicate everything for you. Eventually, you have to be able to talk about yourself and communicate your complexity on dates. Timing and subtlety is important, but watch for opportunities to allude to the fact that you have both a public side and a private side and that your looks and public persona don't tell the full story of who you are.

A guy whose public side is Mr. Traditional but is Mr. Obedient sexually, for example, can tell his date that there is more to him than his straitlaced exterior. This sets the stage for future disclosures about these different parts of your personality. Timing is everything, and you don't want to take the conversation in a sexual direction if it would make your date uncomfortable. But if the mood is right, and there seems to be mutual interest, talking about some of your hidden qualities and interests can help move your relationship forward.

It's possible that Mr. Traditional's date might be interested in and attracted to this side of his personality. Maybe she's secretly Ms. Sinner and a perfect match for his style. But if he never opens the door to this side of himself, there's a chance she'll just assume he's too conservative and too sexually boring for her.

One of the biggest mistakes you can make while you're dating is to pretend to be someone you're not. This is especially true when it comes to sex. If you hide or suppress your sexual persona, and your date does the same, the two of you will never know what your sexual chemistry would really be like if you both let go of your inhibitions.

So if your initial forays into sex are disappointing, you owe it to each other to talk about what really turns you on and the type of sex you secretly long for. As far as you know, he or she may be *exactly* the kind of lover you secretly long for. Maybe she longs to be Ms. Sinner, but she fears you will think she's a slut if she lets that part of her sexuality show. Maybe he's Mr. Dominant, but he is afraid you will think he's a freak if he lets the primitive side of his sexuality show.

What Are Men and Women Most Hesitant to Reveal about Their Sexual Interests?

There's a strange schism in how we talk about sex in our society. People seem to talk about sex and joke about it all the time with their friends. It's a common topic of talk shows, reality shows, and movies. Yet sex is still a taboo topic of conversation in some of the contexts where it matters most.

Dating couples rarely talk about sex before they have it. And after sex, both of them are more likely to talk about the experience with their friends than with each other.

So if I were to make one magical decree about dating that everyone would have to follow, it would be to *talk* about sex with the person you're dating *before* you have sex. Ideally, you would talk about sex afterward too.

Talk about what you enjoy doing sexually. Talk about your favorite sexual activities and positions. But most important, talk about *how* you like to have sex. Talk about the types of sensations, the pace, and the emotional connection that turns you on.

The best way to get this conversation going is to ask questions. Start by asking your date if it would be okay if the two of you talked about sex. If you're a guy, you probably need to reassure your date that you're not using this as a way to initiate sex. Let her know that you're genuinely interested in learning about her sexual desires and what she likes about sex before the two of you take this step physically.

Of the three sexual dimensions, I think the easiest one to talk about is the activity dimension. Ask your date whether he or she likes sex that is fast and intense or slow and sensual or a combination of both. Most people appreciate that both types of sensations can be pleasurable. Liking a slow pace versus a fast pace doesn't make you a bad person. It's a matter of taste.

Unfortunately, people tend to be more judgmental when it comes to the other two dimensions: emotion and power. Men and women with sexual personas on the darker end of the sexual spectrum tend to be especially hesitant to talk about this side of their sexuality. People who are turned on by sex that is dark, naughty, and sinful often feel ashamed about their interests and are afraid they'll be judged harshly or be rejected if they talk about these desires. So if your interests lie in the dark emotional zone, you need to give yourself and your potential partner permission to explore this aspect of sexuality without judgment.

There are even more taboos surrounding power and sex. Even though power plays a role in most people's sexual fantasies and their ideal sexual connection, most men and women are hesitant to talk about the sexual dynamic they find most exciting. Folks who enjoy playing a dominant role will hold themselves back. People who enjoy surrendering are afraid to let go or feel like they should take the lead.

Sometimes when the chemistry is right, these roles just seem to click. You read each other's body language, and everything just seems to fall into place. But it's unrealistic to expect great sex to just happen naturally. Great sex doesn't always just happen. Especially when it comes to issues of power, dominance, and submission, fears and false expectations can easily get in the way.

So talk about what you like, and ask your partner to describe the role he or she finds most exciting and natural. If that doesn't work, experiment with playing different roles. See how your partner responds when you take charge, then give him or her the reins and see how the connection works when you surrender control.

In the next chapter, we'll look at several advanced strategies for exploring forbidden sexual topics. We'll see how talking about your sexual fantasies and sexual role-play can help you improve your sexual chemistry or realign your connection if your sexual spark has fizzled.

Chapter 12

Improving Your Sexual Chemistry within a Relationship

Misaligned Chemistry

Do You Have a Surface Problem or a Deeper Problem?

Over half of the married couples I interviewed said they were disappointed with their sex lives. Some couples say they've lost their sexual spark. They no longer enjoy the same sexual chemistry they had when they first met. Other couples say there has always been something "off" about their sexual connection.

So I am often asked: can a couple reignite their sexual spark?

I believe you can. It's not easy, and it will require both of you to step outside of your comfort zones. But if you're willing to roll up your sleeves and put some time and energy into it, I believe you can dramatically improve and enhance your sexual chemistry.

The first thing you need to do is accept that the loss of your sexual spark is a very common situation faced by many couples. Neither of you are to blame for getting into this situation, but both of you need to take responsibility for finding a way out.

The second thing you need to do is try to disentangle whether your problems are due to differences in sex drive or sexual interests versus a deeper disconnect in sexual chemistry. Back in Chapter 4, we looked at several things you can do if you want sex more or less often than your partner. We also looked at strategies for expanding the variety of your sexual repertoire if one or both of you are feeling bored sexually.

If you and your partner still enjoy a good sexual connection but disagree about how often you have sex or how often you mix up your sexual menu, then you should focus your energy on these relatively straightforward issues. The challenges we'll tackle in this chapter are much deeper issues. If the sexual spark has fizzled, and your sexual chemistry is off, then the two of you are going to be unhappy no matter how often you have sex or what you do sexually.

If this describes your situation, then it's important to recognize that there is a deeper misalignment the two of you have to deal with. It's always a good idea to address basic or surface issues (like the frequency of sex and sexual variety) first, and see if that puts you back on track. But if your sexual spark has fizzled, at least one of you and probably both of you are going to have to try out new sexual roles and news ways of approaching sex.

What Does It Mean to Have Good or Bad Sexual Chemistry?

As I mapped out in the previous chapters, I believe that good sexual chemistry occurs when a couple has sexual personas that fit and match with each other. Ideally, the couple shares a similar emotional approach to sex (light and wholesome versus dark and naughty) and a similar sexual intensity (slow and sensual versus fast and intense) and has a compatible power dynamic (one is more dominant and the other is more submissive or both are versatile).

Sexual chemistry tends to be off when there is a mismatch between the couple's sexual personas. He may enjoy sex that is wholesome and light, but she is drawn to sex that is dark and sinful. He's turned on by tender, affectionate play, while she likes it wild and rough. Both partners may enjoy playing a passive role and wish the other person would take the lead. Both may enjoy being dominant and get frustrated that their partner never fully surrenders sexually. In other words, there are lots of ways that two people's sexual style can conflict and pull in opposing directions.

How Can Your Sexual Chemistry Become Misaligned?

Couples who say there was always something off about their sexual connection can usually trace the source of their disconnect back to the misfit between their sexual personas. If you and your partner started with great sexual chemistry, but then lost it over time, I expect the source of the problem probably has something to do with changes in one or both of your sexual personas.

Let's look at how several personal and relationship developments can potentially alter a couple's sexual personas. Meet Ted and Louise. Ted's sexual persona is Mr. Playful, and Louise is Ms. Romance. They both share a positive and active approach to sex. He enjoys taking charge sexually, and she enjoys surrendering. Since their styles fit, they start their marriage with great sexual chemistry.

Ted and Louise married young, so they both do a fair amount of growing up together and as individuals over the years. Louise gains more confidence as she advances in her career and becomes more assertive. These personality changes carry over into her sexual style. She now takes on a more powerful sexual style and becomes Ms. Passion (positive, dominant, and active). Her husband, Mr. Playful, is proud of her career accomplishments, but he isn't sure how to connect sexually with a partner who is not submissive.

Now, let's imagine a scenario where Louise stays the same, but Ted changes. As Ted matures, he becomes more interested in the darker or more forbidden aspects of sex. His style is now more focused on sex that is dark, naughty, and sinful. So now he fits in the Mr. Dominant category (dark, dominant, and fast). If his wife is uncomfortable with this darker style, then they can become misaligned in several ways. She may still want him to play a dominant role, but not in the rough, wild, or primitive way that is expressed by his new sexual persona.

Perhaps Ted goes through an even bigger transformation. His job involves a lot of pressure and stress. He starts to turn to sex as a way to release stress and temporarily escape from being responsible and in control. So his style morphs into Mr. Sinner (dark, submissive, and fast). Now, the only dimension where he and his wife can connect is their active sexual style. Since she doesn't like darker sexual experiences and doesn't want to play a dominant role, their sexual interests have shifted far apart.

Can Parenting Change Your Chemistry?

If Louise and Ted have kids, there's a good chance that parenting will also change how they see themselves and each other. Over the past two decades, more than twenty-five separate studies have established that marital quality and sexual satisfaction drop, often dramatically, after the transition to parenthood. Couples spend less time together and face more and more pressures and responsibilities.

Based on what I've seen, it looks like kids turn their parents into crazy people. I have a wonderful nephew and three lovely nieces, and a couple of times each year I spend about a week with them. During the first several days of each visit, I am the perfect uncle. However, after a few days, my sanity starts to slip, my patience shrinks, and my fuse gets shorter. By the fifth day, I start saying things like, "Stop it. Stop it! Stopitstopitstopitstopitstopit!" So I won't pretend to know what it's like for a couple to have kids and try to continue to be the sane, charming people they were when they first met.

Even the positive aspects of parenting can change how you see each other. You each take on a new role and identity. Your wife is now a mother. Your husband is now a daddy. Seeing each other in these roles can enhance your *love* for each other, but it may not enhance your sexual attraction.

Being a parent can make it difficult to see yourself or each other as sexual beings. It's hard to be Ms. Affection in the bedroom when you haven't slept in a year and have baby spit-up in your hair. It's hard to be Mr. Discipline in the bedroom after spending an evening being an arbitrator and disciplinarian with your kids.

What Is Your Current Sexual Style?

Regardless of how you got there, it's important to recognize where your current sexual style is centered. Flip back to the exercises in Chapter 10 and identify your sexual persona based on your current sexual interests. Focus on what excites you and turns you on *now*, not what you used to be drawn to.

Has your sexual persona changed over time? Do you think your partner's sexual persona has changed? If so, then I recommend you talk with each other about how your interests have changed.

Remember that change is a natural part of every relationship. You went into the relationship knowing you would have to grow and adapt with each other. Now's the time to step up to the plate and show you can adapt as a couple and become reacquainted with your new sexual selves.

Expanding Your Sexual Style

What Style Would Turn Your Partner On?

Ideally, both of you would make efforts to find common sexual ground and try out new sexual roles. But if someone needs to get the ball rolling, it might as well be you.

Take a look at Exercise 1. The goal of this exercise is to explore the type of emotions, power, and intensity that your partner would

Exercise 1: How to Expand Your Sexual Style

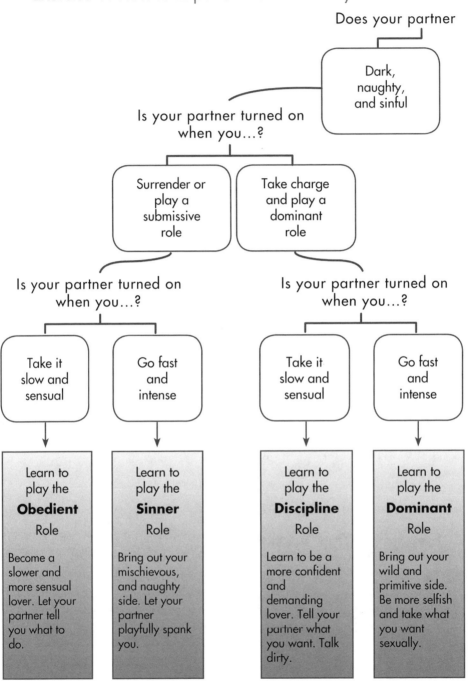

Does your partner

Dark, naughty, and sinful

Is your partner turned on when you...?

Surrender or play a submissive role

Take charge and play a dominant role

Is your partner turned on when you...?

Take it slow and sensual

Go fast and intense

Is your partner turned on when you...?

Take it slow and sensual

Go fast and intense

Learn to play the **Obedient** Role

Become a slower and more sensual lover. Let your partner tell you what to do.

Learn to play the **Sinner** Role

Bring out your mischievous, and naughty side. Let your partner playfully spank you.

Learn to play the **Discipline** Role

Learn to be a more confident and demanding lover. Tell your partner what you want. Talk dirty.

Learn to play the **Dominant** Role

Bring out your wild and primitive side. Be more selfish and take what you want sexually.

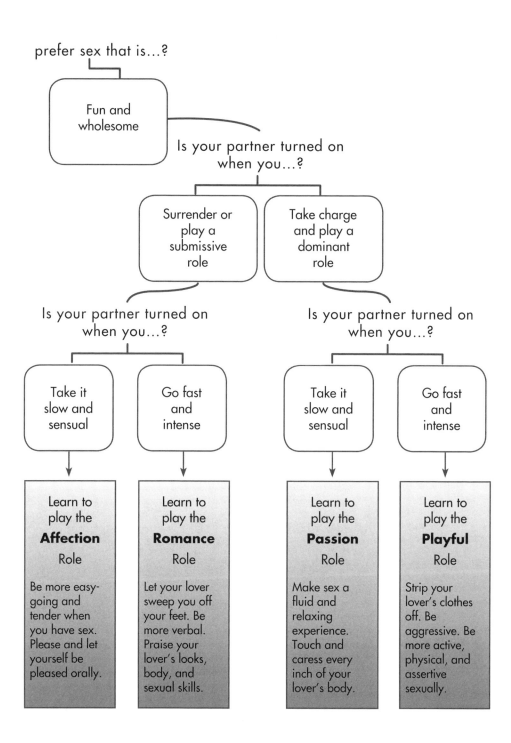

prefer sex that is...?

Fun and wholesome

Is your partner turned on when you...?

Surrender or play a submissive role

Take charge and play a dominant role

Is your partner turned on when you...?

Is your partner turned on when you...?

Take it slow and sensual

Go fast and intense

Take it slow and sensual

Go fast and intense

Learn to play the **Affection** Role

Be more easy-going and tender when you have sex. Please and let yourself be pleased orally.

Learn to play the **Romance** Role

Let your lover sweep you off your feet. Be more verbal. Praise your lover's looks, body, and sexual skills.

Learn to play the **Passion** Role

Make sex a fluid and relaxing experience. Touch and caress every inch of your lover's body.

Learn to play the **Playful** Role

Strip your lover's clothes off. Be aggressive. Be more active, physical, and assertive sexually.

find most exciting. This is your guide to becoming a better lover for your partner.

Ideally, this is something you and your partner can talk about. Ask your partner what he or she would like you to do more of and less of. If talking about it isn't an option or hits a brick wall, approach this like an experiment. At each branching point in the exercise, try approaching sex both ways and see which one sparks the most sexual excitement.

The branches in Exercise 1 should point you toward a sexual persona that will be compatible with your partner's style. If you can learn to embody this persona and enjoy it, then the two of you should enjoy great sexual chemistry again.

The exercise ends with a brief recommendation for expanding your sexual style. Let's take a closer look at how you can make a few of these deeper shifts and become more comfortable with different sexual zones.

How Can I Make Sex More Playful and Fun?

Sex can take a variety of forms, each with a different emotional flavor. Sex can be serious and profound, like when you connect with someone on a deep and intimate level. It can be dark and primitive, like when you explore the Kinky topics we'll look at in a moment. But sex can also be light, carefree, and fun.

A surprising number of men and women find it difficult to approach sex in a playful and fun way. I say it's surprising because I think sex is supposed to be fun. We're biologically programmed to find sex pleasurable. Sex feels good in lots of different ways. It can be exciting and arousing, and then calming and relaxing.

Of course, sex can have serious consequences. It can lead to pregnancy. There are sexually transmitted diseases to worry about. It brings up a lot of religious and moral prohibitions. So it's understandable that many of us learned to associate sex with very serious thoughts and emotions. For a lot of folks, sex has rarely been carefree or easy.

But if you want to rekindle your sexual spark, learning to approach sex in a playful way is extremely important. If you are going to expand your sexual style and invite your partner to expand his or her style, you are going to have to create an environment where you can try new things, act in new ways, and feel new emotions, without being scrutinized or judged.

Start by thinking about a hobby or favorite activity where you find it easy to have fun and play. Maybe it's cooking, gardening, hiking, playing sports, or watching sports. Think about the mind-set you bring to this activity. What do you do that gives yourself permission to play? Most people say their playtime is unpressured and carefree. It's a time when they can just go with the flow and be themselves.

This is the attitude and energy you want to bring to sex. You can't force yourself to have fun, but you can *allow* yourself to have fun. You can choose to let go of the normal structure and expectations that make sex the same each time. You can allow yourself to be silly and open to trying new things.

A playful approach to sex can open the door to experiencing either end of the emotional continuum. Playful sex can be light and wholesome, but it can also open the door to darker, primitive play. Letting go of rules and structure can let you be fun and silly or wild and animalistic. It's up to you.

How Can I Be a More Sensual Lover?

Most women (and some men) say they wished their partner would slow sex down and be more sensual lovers. There's nothing wrong with fast and intense sex, but great lovers know how to shift between multiple gears. They can take it slow, then crank it up, and then slow it down again.

So ask yourself: What's the rush? Where is the need for speed coming from?

For men, these fast habits are often carryovers from masturbation. For most men, masturbation is a no-nonsense, utilitarian exercise. It's something we learned to do quickly and quietly. So many men gravitate toward fast movements and tight and strong sensations out of force of habit. It's always gotten the job done during solo sex, so it seems natural to take that approach with a partner.

Most women approach masturbation quite differently from men. Women's bodies tend to take a little longer to warm up. Fast and intense sensations play a part, but it's not where most women start when they're pleasing themselves.

If masturbation played a role in causing this disconnect, I think it can play a role in readjusting your styles. For men, I recommend incorporating slower and softer sensations into your masturbation routine. Consider it homework! Show your body that it can enjoy a different approach to arousal and then carryover these new skills to sex with your partner.

I also recommend that you practice masturbating together. This is a useful experience for both men and women, but especially for men. If you're a guy, ask your partner to masturbate while you hold her or just watch. Pay attention to how she touches herself, the pace of her movements, and how she varies the intensity and strength of the sensations. Next time, ask if you can stimulate her while she guides you with her hands.

This will also help you expand the amount of foreplay the two of you incorporate into sex. Couples with very fast sexual styles tend to skip over oral sex and manual stimulation and rush into intercourse. I'd recommend you take a break from intercourse or at least focus more of your sexual energy on other activities in your sexual repertoire.

Being a more sensual lover means expanding the senses that you call upon during sex. It means exciting multiple body zones and not just the penis and vagina. As a start, I recommend you kiss twice as much. Spend twice as much time playing with each other's nipples. Massage and stroke each other's bodies twice as much as you usually do.

Finally, in order to approach sex at a slower pace, you're both going to need to adjust your expectations about erections. One of the most common myths about male physiology is that a "normal" healthy man stays firmly erect throughout sex. In fact, studies have found that the average man loses and regains his erection three or four times during intercourse.[45]

As you focus more of your sexual energy on foreplay and slow down the speed and intensity of sex, these cycles of being firmly erect, then softer, then erect again are going to be even more frequent. Some guys would rather play fast and hard with their initial erection than risk the frustration and embarrassment of losing their erection. So it's important that you both talk about this and give the guy permission not to have a constant raging erection during every moment of sex.

Why Should You Have More Quickies?

If you're already comfortable with the slow and sensual side of sex, you may want to expand your skills on the other end of the continuum. Great lovers know how to bring a primitive, passionate, and out-of-control energy to sex.

To practice this side of your sexuality, I recommend you and your partner have more quickies. Sex in loving, long-term relationships tends to fall into routines of mutual satisfaction. Quickies mix things up by introducing spontaneity and selfishness back into sex.

Quickies don't have to be planned. You can fit them into any ten-minute window when you're both in the mood. Quickies also let you focus on getting your needs met in the fastest and most efficient way possible.

Sexual Role-Play

How Can Sexual Role-Play Improve Your Sex Life?

Sexual role-play can be a great way to expand your sexual style. Lots of couples use role-play to explore their sexual fantasies and incorporate new kinds of emotions into sex.

Role-play can also help you try out new ways to relate to each other sexually. If you and your partner have a preferred power dynamic, role-play can help you break out of your old habits. If your partner wants you to be more dominant or more submissive than comes naturally to you, role-play can help you try out this new dynamic.

There are several levels of role-play. There's the basic level. Let's call it role-play "light," where you define your roles verbally. It's informal and playful (like he's the quarterback, and she's the cheerleader). Then there's advanced role-play, where you plan ahead, have clearly defined roles and scripts; maybe you meet somewhere outside of the house, or at least have sex outside of the bedroom. Some couples use costumes or props to add to the effect.

A lot of men and women are comfortable with light role-play, but they are intimidated by more advanced scenarios or costumes. But I encourage you to shake things up and be willing to step outside of your comfort zone.

Coincidentally, I'm writing this on Halloween. It's always been one of my favorite holidays. I love seeing kids dressed up and having fun. But I also enjoy seeing adults being silly and letting their creative and goofy sides run free. I think most couples would benefit from bringing some of this same energy into their sex lives. Whether it's Halloween or Mardi Gras, there's something freeing and exciting about putting on a costume or mask and assuming a new identity.

To give you some ideas, let's look at some of the most popular role-play scenarios among both men and women. Then we'll see how you can use fantasies and role-play to realign your sexual chemistry with your partner.

What Role-Play Scenarios Have You Tried or Would You Be Open to Trying?

To identify men and women's favorite role-play scenarios, I conducted several studies. As part of the study of sexual fantasies that

I described in Chapter 9, I asked men and women whether they had ever acted out their fantasies as part of sexual role-play with a partner. For those who said yes, I asked them to describe what they did and the roles they and their partners played. Then I took the twenty most common scenarios and asked another large sample of men and women to rate how interested they would be in trying out each scenario with their partner.[46]

What Are Women's Favorite Role-Play Scenarios?

The four most popular role-play scenarios among women cover a range of emotions and power dynamics. Some women enjoyed light and wholesome versions of the scenarios, while other women enjoyed darker and edgier versions.

1. *Pretend to be strangers.*

   This is one of the most popular scenarios among both women and men. It's also one of the easiest and most straightforward to try out.

   The couple picks a bar or coffee shop to meet at. They pretend to be strangers who meet, seduce each other, and then go home or to a motel for no-strings-attached sex.

   Some couples maintain their own identities. Others like to pretend to be different people.

   Most women enjoy the romance of connecting again for the first time. They enjoy the attention, the eye contact, and the spontaneity of being swept off their feet.

2. *Encounter with a masked intruder.*

   This scenario falls on the darker end of the fantasy continuum. It plays with fantasies about force and shakes up the power dynamics in the relationship.

   She pretends to be home alone and asleep in bed.

He sneaks into bed with his clothes on (the ski mask is optional) and surprises her. The couple decides up front whether they want to have a pretend struggle or incorporate a specific dialogue.

This is obviously a scenario where the couple has to have a very trusting relationship and must talk up front about their comfort zones and limits. With all such scenarios, it is also important to have a *safe word,* which both partners understand to mean that they stop immediately, quit the role-play, and talk.

3. *She plays a call girl.*

The idea of playing a call girl was appealing to a number of women. They liked the idea of being desired and lusted after. It also takes sex out of the loving emotional realm into a playful or naughty world.

This is a fantasy that, in a twisted way, gives both partners a chance to be dominant and in control. As the call girl, she decides what's on the sexual menu and how much each act costs. Her partner gets to pick what he wants. This frees both partners from the ridiculous expectation that you instinctively know what each other wants or can read each other's mind.

Maybe she surprises him by putting a few adventurous items on the menu that are not normally available. Maybe he surprises her by picking a couple of items that he knows she enjoys, but that rarely get included in their sexual routine.

Most women said they would want to play a sophisticated and high-priced call girl. But some were more turned on by playing a prostitute or streetwalker. One couple said they routinely meet at a sleazy hotel. He pretends to be a corrupt cop, and she pretends to be a streetwise hooker.

4. *Getting it on with her plumber.*

Sex with a plumber or other repairman is a common sexual fantasy and the fourth most popular role-play scenario among women.

She plays a housewife. He plays a butch repairman invited in to check out her plumbing. The two of them have to squeeze into tight places, check out the pipes under the sink, or maybe there's a problem with the shower, which "accidentally" sprays them with water. Regardless of the exact scenario, there's always lots of fun plumbing talk and sexual innuendo.

Women described both light, fun versions of this scenario and darker versions. Some women prefer to play a naive housewife who is seduced or even overpowered by the repairman. Other women prefer to be the sexual aggressor who seduces the innocent repairman.

What Are Men's Favorite Role-Play Scenarios?

All of the scenarios I just described were also popular among men. Three additional role-play scenarios stand out as particularly appealing to men.

1. *Tie him up.*

About half of all men say they fantasize about being dominated by a powerful and dark female figure. So it's not surprising that the most popular role-play scenario among men puts their partner in a dominant role and involves being tied up and blindfolded.

His hands are tied together with something soft (like an old scarf or tube socks), or if it's a darker fantasy, something rough (rope or nonlocking handcuffs). Some men like to be tied to the bedposts and maybe even have both arms and legs tied.

Many men said they liked being tied up because it was strangely freeing. He's freed from expectations to perform. He's not expected to move or act or make decisions. He has to surrender control to his partner. He plays a passive role like a pupil, pet, or slave.

Meanwhile, this role empowers her to take charge in a way that most women rarely feel comfortable doing otherwise. She's free to do what she wants at her own pace.

If she's playing a dominatrix, she also folds discipline and punishment into the play. She shouts her commands, and if he resists, she lightly spanks or paddles him. A little pain heightens his sensations and enhances her power.

As noted above, such role-play requires planning and a frank discussion up front. Since bondage often turns into a game where no can mean yes, you need a neutral safe word (like pumpkin or Palestine) that means stop.

2. *He's a Don Juan.*

The next most popular role-play scenario among men is actually a collection of several fantasy scenarios that lets the man play a perfect lover and seducer. In all these scenarios the woman plays an innocent and passive role (a nurse, princess, or virgin bride). Her job is to be seduced and overwhelmed by the passionate advances of her partner.

The man gets to play the irresistible playboy or Don Juan. He's sexually assertive and very verbal about what he wants and what he wants to do to her sexually.

These roles can be played out in the bedroom. Or you can incorporate the seduction into the scenario I described earlier, where the couple pretends to be strangers and meets at a bar or coffee shop.

3. *She does a striptease.*

The next most popular role-play scenario among men involves having their partner do a striptease or lap dance for them, while he plays a stranger or out-of-town businessman.

Several couples described similar scenarios where the man sits in a chair in the middle of the room while his partner strips and dances to sexy music. She enters wearing her sexiest lingerie under a jacket or trench coat. Then she unwraps herself slowly, layer by layer.

Since the rules require that he not touch her, she runs her hands all over her body and touches herself in ways that he longs to touch her. She flirts, throws her hair around, and makes sideways glances. She tempts and teases him until he can't bear it any longer.

Why Is Sexual Role-Play So Powerful?

I'm a big fan of sexual role-play as a way to rekindle sexual chemistry. Of all the tools and ideas in this book, I think talking about your sexual fantasies with your partner and then acting them out through role-play have the biggest potential to transform your sex life and reignite your sexual spark.

Part of this magic comes from the power of being understood at a deep, instinctual level. Most of us grew up keeping our sexual desires wrapped up in secrets and shame. It's a rare and wonderful experience to have a partner who genuinely wants to understand your sexual desires.

So ask your partner about his or her fantasies. Find a time when you are both relaxed and comfortable and take turns describing some of your fantasies. If you're nervous, start off with safe fantasies. Talk about simple scenes and scenarios that turn you on. Show your partner that you can listen to his or her fantasies without judgment or criticism. Ask questions ("Then what happens?"). Help your partner paint a picture of the situation, his or her feelings, and what happens at each stage of the fantasy.

Once the two of you are comfortable in talking about your fantasies, you may want to try out some of the exercises in Chapter 9. Take turns circling fantasy characters, settings, and actions that turn you on. See if you're both drawn to similar fantasy zones or to different zones.

Then take the next step and find ways to act out some of your favorite fantasies. If you both enjoy being verbal as part of sex, role-play can start by simply saying who each of you want to be ("I'm the coach...who are you?"). You can describe the scene as you go along. Or you can do a little planning ahead of time and map out the scenario before you dive in.

Can You Use Role-Play to Make Specific Adjustments?

I recommend using role-play to try out new approaches to sex and new ways of connecting, without agendas or expectations. But it's also possible to use role-play as a way to make specific adjustments to your sexual dynamics. If your sexual personas have changed over time or become misaligned, you can use role-play to try out new personas.

It's not uncommon for men to have a hard time turning off their dominant side, for example. That's why the "tie me up" scenario or the stripper scenario can be freeing for both partners. The role gives him permission to relax and let his partner take control, and it gives her permission to touch and be touched and to set the pace and intensity she enjoys.

Great lovers have the ability to transport their partner away from the drudgery of day-to-day life and into a world of possibility. Role-play gives both you and your partner this power. It's a great way to take your relationship away from the limits and pressures of your day-to-day lives and remind each other that there is something deep and instinctual that still connects you.

Conclusion

I saved one of my favorite questions about sex for last. I have a very unscientific theory that your answer to this question offers unique insights into your sexual history and your approach to sex throughout your life. Here's the question: when and how did you first learn about sex and what was your reaction to this news?

I first heard about sex when I was eight years old. The messenger just so happened to be my girlfriend at the time, and she was eager to share what she had learned from an enlightening conversation with her parents the night before. As we were riding home on the school bus, she told me and my best friend, Eddie, in graphic detail, how sex works.

Frankly, both Eddie and I were shocked. When she was through describing the mechanics of sexual intercourse, I remember saying, "I think you're making this up, but if you're telling the truth, it sounds like a really *weird* thing to do."

I've asked hundreds of people to describe how they first learned about sex, and every story has been unique. The emotional reactions have ranged from shock and disgust to fascination and exhilaration. Yet there's one theme that runs through all the stories I've heard, and that's the curiosity that all kids bring to the idea of sex. Kids are curious about sex before they learn the details, and the first bits of news spark even greater curiosity.

Most of us start out curious about the mechanics of sex. When I was thirteen, my eccentric Aunt Billie smuggled me a copy of the 1969 classic *Everything You Always Wanted to Know about Sex (But Were Afraid to Ask)*.[47] Apparently, back then, the big mysteries about sex centered on differences in male and female physiology, sexual response, and sexual technique. These are still interesting topics (and there are now shelves filled with books on these issues). But now, forty years later, the real mysteries about sex and the questions we are most afraid to ask have less to do with *what* sex is than the *who* and the *how* of making sex a fun and satisfying part of our lives and relationships.

I wrote this book to share what I've learned over the past decade as I studied the sex lives of men and women online. I've taken a close look at the features and qualities that men and women find most and least attractive. I've also examined the wide variety of sexual desires and interests men and women bring to their relationships. In the end, my answer to whom you should sleep with has to do with finding two keys to sexual compatibility.

The first key, as we explored in Parts 1 and 2, has to do with basic sexual logistics. If you're single, I recommend finding a partner who has a similar sex drive and similar interests in sexual variety. As we saw in Part 1, the good news for single men and women is that there are plenty of men and women with every combination of sexual tastes.

What's also fortunate is that there are very similar numbers of men and women with *high* sex drives. More women than men have Vanilla sexual tastes, and slightly more men than women have Adventurous or Kinky tastes. But these differences are not huge. So, in theory, there's no reason why every man or woman with a high sex drive and adventurous taste shouldn't be able to find a partner with similar interests. Since most men and women have low to moderate sex drives and Mainstream sexual tastes, there should be lots of potential matches for these folks as well.

Yet the real world doesn't always work as you expect it would in theory. In the real world, sexual interests often remain hidden from ourselves and each other. Questions about how often you like to have sex and how adventurous you want your sex life to be rarely get discussed during the dating process. So, many couples become emotionally connected and start to form relationships before they consider whether or not they fit together sexually.

That's why we also explored in Chapter 4 ways to talk about where your sex drives and interests overlap (or differ) and how to find common ground that will satisfy both of your needs. In this way, one of the surprising answers to "who should you have sex with" is this: pick someone who cares about your needs and is willing to make compromises. Men and women who manage to keep their natural curiosity about sex alive and are willing to explore their own desires and their partner's desires tend to make the best long-term lovers even if the initial fit in sex drives and adventurousness is imperfect.

Back when I first started designing matchmaking systems for Match.com and Yahoo!, I believed that matching based on similar sex drives and interests in sexual variety would ensure sexual compatibility. At the time, folding sexual interests into mainstream matchmaking was controversial and (in my opinion) a big step forward. But over time, as I followed up on which matches worked out and which did not, it became clear to me that these "basics" of sexual compatibility were only part of the story.

That's why the second part of my answer to "who should you sleep with" centers on the importance of sexual chemistry. It's possible for a couple to be attracted to each other, have similar sex drives, and even enjoy the same sexual activities and yet still have no chemistry in the bedroom. My research into these bedroom surprises is what opened my eyes to the differences between our public personalities and our private sexual personalities.

Ideally, you should find a partner whose sexual persona fits with your own. So, in Part 3, we learned about the three core ingredients of sexual chemistry. We explored whether you were drawn to sex that is wholesome and fun or nasty and naughty. We explored whether you were turned on by sex that is fast and intense or slow and sensual. We even explored the taboo topic of power and sex and whether you like to take charge during sex or surrender and lose control.

We saw how these three dimensions express themselves in your fantasy life and how your sexual fantasies offer a window into your deepest sexual desires and fears. They show us what you want sex to be as well as highlight the obstacles that stand in your way.

Then we saw how these ingredients combine to create your unique sexual persona and how you can use these dimensions to understand the sexual style of your current or future lover. My research suggests that there are sizable numbers of men and women with each of the sexual personas. Even an individual with the rarest style shares his or her approach with at least one in ten men and women.

The proportion of men and women who have a dark, sinful, and naughty approach to sex is very similar (about one in three). Most women have a gentler and more submissive sexual style, but at least one in three like to play a strong, forceful, and dominant role sexually. Meanwhile, men are almost equally divided in their approach to power and sex; about half want to play a dominant role while the other half enjoy playing a more submissive role.

So, again, in theory, there is no reason why single men and women shouldn't be able to find partners with compatible sexual personas. Yet, in the real world, I realize this is often easier said than done. Although I intended the information in Part 3 to be empowering, I realize some of you will probably find it overwhelming.

Many early readers told me they enjoyed learning this new sexual vocabulary and were relieved to have a framework that helped them understand why they clicked with some partners but clashed with others. However, other readers have told me they felt discouraged by learning "all the ways that things can go wrong." Maybe you're like one reader who told me, "Ignorance is bliss." Or maybe you're like Han Solo, who said, "Never tell me the odds!"

But as we saw in Part 4, there's no need to feel hopeless or helpless. If you're single, knowing about sexual personas can help you clarify whom you are searching for and whom you want to avoid. Knowing the external traits to watch for as clues to a potential partner's sexual persona (like shyness, intelligence, and rebelliousness) can also save you time and energy.

If you're in a relationship, knowing how to explore your sexual fantasies and incorporate some of them into sexual role-play can open up new ways of connecting and reignite your sexual spark. Maybe you'll try out one of the seven popular role-play scenarios that I described in Chapter 12, or maybe you'll find another way to adjust your sexual style to surprise and excite your partner.

In the end, your ability to turn all this information into something useful depends almost entirely on your willingness to talk about the ingredients of sexual chemistry with your current (or future) partner. Hopefully, this book has given you a new vocabulary and new questions and tools you can use to explore what you and your partner truly desire sexually. Whether you're single or already in a relationship, I believe it's never too late to reignite your sexual spark, and it's never too late to have a great sex life.

Endnotes

Chapter 1: Sex Drive

1. The parts of the brain that run through the lateral hypo-
   thalamus to the limbic system and forebrain are part of the
   self-stimulation system of the brain. This area is also associated with addiction. In animal studies, electrical stimulation
   of this area can cause an animal to search for food or other
   desired objects persistently to the point of exhaustion.

2. The trends summarized in this chapter and the next
   combine the findings from several large studies where we
   recruited from two large Web portals. In total, the research
   I reference here is based on surveys of 3,254,012 men and
   3,890,233 women. The samples are largely representative of
   Internet users in terms of age, race, income, education, and
   geographic location.

3. We have examined responses to questions about desired sexual frequency and sex drive in over ten million men and over twelve million women.

Chapter 2: Sexual Variety

4. The most popular meal in 1954 was referenced in Weiss, *The Clustered World.*

5. Dr. Kinsey was an entomologist by training and had done years of field research cataloging five million varieties of gall wasps. So when he took it upon himself to do what no one in history had ever done before—that is, ask people from all walks of life about their sexual behaviors—he used a similar field research methodology. He started by driving out to the small farms around Bloomington and gathered sexual histories from the farm workers, each of which he recorded on a single index card. Eventually, he personally gathered over eleven thousand such cards from men and women.

6. A young person at a recent lecture raised his hand and argued that among his generation the meaning of the bases has changed. He proceeded to inform us of the new base landmarks. Let me just say, I don't know what kind of ball you kids are playing, but it is *not* baseball!

7. Some individuals go through periods in their lives when they become restless and easily bored with sex and life in general. Men going through a stereotypic midlife crisis, for example, often seek out clothes, cars, and sometimes new sexual partners or experiences in an attempt to feel young and vigorous again.

8. It's worth noting that this is one of the few findings for which there were strong racial differences. The trend of one in four adults seeking a more adventurous partner is a very Caucasian phenomenon. This trend is virtually absent among African Americans, for example, who consistently prefer a partner with similar sexual tastes.

Chapter 3: Clues That Reveal Sexual Compatibility

9. See Gottman, *Why Marriages Succeed or Fail*, for how this has been noted across his studies.

10. For reviews, see Gottman and Krokoff, "The Relationship between Marital Interaction and Marital Satisfaction," and Gottman and Notarius, "Decade Review: Observing Marital Interaction."

11. The poor predictive value of personality tests in predicting long-term marriage success has been noted by Houston and Houts, "The Psychological Infrastructure of Courtship and Marriage," and others. The exception to this may be the independent influence of neuroticism on marital longevity, although it has been questioned whether neuroticism is a proxy for depression, which is known to have a serious impact on marital stability.

12. It is important to distinguish between the nature of screening tests (which are for asymptomatic people) and diagnostic tests (which are calibrated among people already showing a disease, disorder, or problem behavior). Online dating is basically conducting a screening test on a nonexistent relationship to predict its likelihood of

developing into a good marriage or a bad one. False positives outnumber true positives with every screening test in medicine and psychology. Because screening tests are not 100 percent accurate and are performed on pairs of individuals who are unlikely to end up together (i.e., date, get engaged, get married, and then divorced), the risk of a false-positive result is significant. As with all tests, the interpretation of the result depends upon the prevalence of the disorder in the population being tested (Bayes theorem). For example, in a pool of potential dating candidates, let's say 1 percent of all the dates I might meet is a potential divorce (meaning I'd likely want to date this person, marry her, and years later decide to divorce her). This would be the only value of the test, since if I would exclude the remaining people from consideration myself, only this 1 percent is worthy of concern. If the hypothetical divorce detection device has a sensitivity and specificity of 90 percent, the positive predictive value (i.e., the probability of true disease if the screening test is positive) is 8.3 percent. Thus, eleven people will receive false-positive results compared with every true positive (or true potential divorce predicted). This is only a concern if one of the false positives is a person I am very interested in meeting and would be a wonderful match and spouse. Thus, the impact of saving people from negative events has to be balanced with how the false conclusions might change the future in unanticipated ways. False negatives would also be an issue, since such couples would have false reassurance and not take steps to address underlying problems along the way. Although most of us expect we could ignore such findings if we disagreed with them, research suggests that false test results in medicine (such as being inaccurately diagnosed with hypertension or high cholesterol) resulted in lasting disability, even though the false-positive test results were corrected relatively quickly. For further background, see the in-depth mathematical treatments by evidence-based medicine champion Eddy, *Common Screening Tests.*

13. I pulled from multiple studies in determining the popularity of the *public personas.* I've been fortunate to have had the opportunity to study preferences in a variety of settings on the Internet and in the real world. I have studied people planning to get married, others looking to date casually, and some seeking sexual encounters only. For our purposes here, I combined all of this data to offer a broad view of the relative popularity of each persona.

14. We found parallel trends in personality types when we looked at the "Big 5" framework and when using the popular Myers-Briggs type inventory. People with SJ types (described as traditionalists in the Myers-Briggs framework) tend to have lower levels of sexual desire and less adventurousness than those with opposite profiles.

15. The different combinations of *extroversion* (outgoing, active, assertive) and *conscientiousness* (organized, reliable, efficient) are linked to both sexual desire and adventurousness. Mr. or Ms. Shy, who is low in extroversion and high in conscientiousness, is usually less interested in sex than Mr. or Ms. Adventure, who is high in extroversion and low in conscientiousness. I found the same trend when I looked at our research using the Myers-Briggs type inventory (MBTI). Of the sixteen core types, the four IJ types (which translates into high in introversion and high in judgment, which is like conscientiousness) have the lowest levels of sexual desire and sexual adventurousness.

Meanwhile, the four EP types (high in extroversion and high in perception, which is the opposite of conscientiousness) have the highest sexual interests.

16. In the Myers-Briggs studies, high N (intuitive), which captures abstract thinking and imagination, is linked to greater interest in sexual role-play and having more frequent and complex sexual fantasies. The same trend exists looking at openness in the Big Five research.

Chapter 4: Keeping the Spark Alive

17. Ephron, *I Feel Bad about My Neck*.

18. Flaubert, *Madame Bovary*.

19. Most of the women and men in my studies say that fidelity is among the most important things to making a relationship work long term. Few situations can wreak greater emotional havoc than not remaining monogamous. Once the trust in a relationship has been broken, it is usually a long and uphill battle to regain your emotional and sexual connection.

Chapter 5: The Three Ingredients of Sexual Chemistry

20. Across several of my studies, about two out of three men and one in three women said they fantasized about someone other than their regular partner at least once a month. A surprisingly large subgroup of men (about one in four) say they fantasize about someone other than their wife or girlfriend every day. In contrast, less than one in twenty women

say they fantasize about someone other than their husband or boyfriend every day.

21. No one knows for sure why we have sexual fantasies or what function they serve. I'm inclined to view sex as just one of many things we fantasize about. It's one of many topics and targets of our very active imaginations. Imagination helps us anticipate possible situations and mentally practice different actions. We can imagine a variety of possible futures and identify which one we want to pursue. If you can imagine a goal (building a house, dating a supermodel, having a three-way, etc.) and imagine ways of making it happen, it brings you one step closer to achieving it. It's also possible to look at fantasies as waking dreams. Of course, no one knows for sure why we dream or what dreams really mean. The best explanation I have heard is that dreams practice a wide variety of scenarios so that our minds have preexisting neural pathways to put into action in case we encounter rare situations, especially scary ones (like being chased by a lion or showing up at the office in your underwear). Of course, to explain all the time and energy we invest in our internal sex lives, we can always fall back on the same explanation I offered for why we pursue our external sex lives: It feels good! Fantasies are fun. They help us escape from boredom, loneliness, and frustration. We'll look at possible motivations and interpretations of fantasies in Chapter 9.

22. Men and women appear to fantasize for similar reasons but with somewhat different connections to their external sex lives. I've found in my research that men fantasize (and masturbate) more often when they do not have a sexual partner or are not having sex as frequently as they would like. Women's internal sex lives, however, are most active

when their external sex lives are active as well. Women who are in a relationship and/or have a regular sexual partner report having more sexual fantasies than women who do not have a sexual partner. In other words, during sexual dry spells, men tend to make up for limits in their external sex life by creating a richer and more active internal sex life. In contrast, women appear more likely to shut down altogether during periods when they do not have a regular sexual partner.

23. Symbolic interactionism is a theoretical school or orientation in sociological social psychology. For overviews, see Stryker, *Symbolic Interactionism*, and Smith-Lovin and Heise, *Analyzing Social Interaction*. Drs. Stryker and Heise and my fellow graduate students (especially Melissa Milkie, Aileen Schulte, and Erica Sharkansky) in the measurement of affect program at Indiana University contributed greatly to my understanding of these theories and their wide-ranging applications.

24. A toaster, by the way, is a positive, somewhat powerful, and active object.

Chapter 7: Power and Sex

25. Stein, *Lovers, Friends, Slaves...The Nine Male Sexual Types.*

26. For anyone with lingering doubts about the importance and relevance of power dynamics and sex, I recommend Waal's *Our Inner Ape.* He does a wonderful job exploring parallels with our ape cousins. On the topic of power and sex, he notes, "The fundamental difference between our two closest

relatives is that one resolves sexual issues with power, while the other resolves power issues with sex" (p. 18). He's referring to the fact that chimpanzees are very status focused and use power hierarchies to control access to sexual partners. Meanwhile, bonobos use sex as a way of promoting empathy, caring, and cooperation and resolving power conflicts.

27. These estimates of preferred styles were drawn from a series of online studies with a total of 5,433 men and 5,011 women.

Chapter 8: Sex and Intensity

28. Berger et al., *Ways of Seeing*.

29. My research with these images was built on the pioneering research of Peter J. Lang and colleagues at the *Center for the Study of Emotion and Attention* (see Ito, Cacioppo, and Lang, "Eliciting Affect Using the International Affective Picture System"; and Lang, Bradley, and Cuthbert, "Emotion and Motivation").

Chapter 9: Sexual Fantasies

30. The exercises featured here were tested with 511 men and 678 women. They are based on a series of online studies, starting with a study of 417 men and 394 women who wrote about their fantasies in an online survey. This was followed by another online study that asked 1,288 men and 1,019 women to rate the fantasy characters, settings, and actions on the three dimensions featured in this chapter.

31. Bader, *Arousal: The Secret Logic of Sexual Fantasies.*

32. Although I'm sure we didn't evolve these skills in order to have hot sexual fantasies, it is certainly a nice fringe benefit.

33. See, e.g., the compilations of fantasies developed by Nancy Friday, *Beyond My Control, Men in Love,* and *My Secret Garden.*

34. Classical Freudian theory refers to this aspect of character as the dual-instinct theory. It argues that we become turned on by both sex *and* violence.

35. Violence is pervasive in our society. It is also pervasive in storytelling. Even children's stories such as the Three Little Pigs center on violent themes. Our fantasies develop alongside all the other stories we learn. So violence is bound to seep into the plots of our fantasies.

36. Kahr, *Who's Been Sleeping in Your Head?*

37. There are other fantasy devices to work around this obstacle, such as imagining perfect communication during sex, but for many men this may not even be conceivable.

Chapter 10: Sexual Personas

38. See "I contain multitudes," from Walt Whitman's *Leaves of Grass.*

39. For an excellent exploration of the multiple selves theory, see Carter, *Multiplicity.*

40. The full quotation from Ralph Waldo Emerson's 1841 essay on self-reliance: "Foolish consistency is the hobgoblin of little minds." Emerson espoused a belief that everything is to be questioned and that doing the same thing over and over is not a virtue.

41. This is drawn from online surveys of 1,012 men and 1,230 women who rated their own sexual styles on each of these three dimensions and used the descriptive words used in the exercises.

42. This investigation was the second part of the survey mentioned above of 1,012 men and 1,230 women.

Chapter 11: Finding a Sexual Persona That Fits Yours

43. See Cox's *Superdate* and *Superflirt*.

44. Regardless of how well eating, dancing, or hiking predict sexual activity styles, they all serve as good metaphors. There is no right way or wrong way to eat or hike. There are definitely good dancers and bad dancers, but who looks the most ridiculous depends on your own definition of good dancing. The ideal partner in each of these activities has a style that is similar to your own. A compatible dinner companion, for example, eats at a similar pace. If you eat very quickly and your date eats very slowly, you'll either starve to death or be bored to tears before your partner finishes her salad.

Chapter 12: Improving Your Sexual Chemistry within a Relationship

45. See Masters and Johnson, *Human Sexual Inadequacy*, and Masters and Johnson, *Human Sexual Response*.

46. An online survey of 1,453 men and 1,389 women ranked their top twenty favorite sexual fantasies.

Conclusion

47. Reuben, *Everything You Always Wanted to Know about Sex (But Were Afraid to Ask)*.

Bibliography

Bader, Michael J. *Arousal: The Secret Logic of Sexual Fantasies*. New York: St. Martin's Press, 2003.

Berger, John, et al. *Ways of Seeing*. New York: Penguin Books, 1972.

Carter, Rita. *Multiplicity: The New Science of Personality, Identity, and the Self*. New York: Little, Brown, 2008.

Cox, Tracey. *Superdate*. London: DK Ault, 2004.

———. *Superflirt*. London: DK Ault, 2003.

de Waal, Frans B. M. *Our Inner Ape: A Leading Primatologist Explains Why We Are Who We Are*. New York: Penguin Group, 2005.

Eddy, David. M. *Common Screening Tests*. Philadelphia: American College of Physicians, 1991.

Ephron, Nora. *I Feel Bad about My Neck: And Other Thoughts on Being a Woman*. New York: Knopf, 2006.

Flaubert, Gustave. *Madame Bovary*. 1857. Reprint, New York: Penguin Classics, 2002.

Friday, Nancy. *Beyond My Control: Forbidden Fantasies in an Uncensored Age*. Naperville, IL: Sourcebooks, 2009.

_____. *Men in Love: Men's Sexual Fantasies*. New York: Delta, 1998.

_____. *My Secret Garden: Women's Sexual Fantasies*. New York: Pocket, 2008.

Gottman, John M. *Why Marriages Succeed or Fail: What You Can Learn from the Breakthrough Research to Make Your Marriage Last*. New York: Simon & Schuster, 1994.

Gottman, John M., and L. J. Krokoff. "The Relationship between Marital Interaction and Marital Satisfaction: A Longitudinal View." *Journal of Consulting and Clinical Psychology* 57 (1989): 47–52.

Gottman, John M., and C. I. Notarius. "Decade Review: Observing Marital Interaction." *Journal of Marriage and the Family* 62, no. 4 (2000): 927–47.

Houston, T. L., and R. M. Houts. "The Psychological Infrastructure of Courtship and Marriage: The Role of Personality and Compatibility in Romantic Relationships." In *The Developmental Course of Marital Dysfunction*, edited by Thomas N. Bradbury. New York: Cambridge University Press, 1998.

Ito, T. A., J. T. Cacioppo, and Peter J. Lang. "Eliciting Affect Using the International Affective Picture System: Trajectories through Evaluative Space." *Society for Personality and Social Psychology* 24 (1998): 855–79.

Kahr, Brett. *Who's Been Sleeping in Your Head? The Secret World of Sexual Fantasies*. New York: Basic Books, 2009.

Lang, Peter J., M. M. Bradley, and B. N. Cuthbert. "Emotion and Motivation: Measuring Affective Perception." *Journal of Clinical Neurophysiology* 15 (1998): 397–408.

Masters, William H., and Virginia E. Johnson. *Human Sexual Inadequacy.* Boston: Little, Brown, 1970.

_____. *Human Sexual Response.* Boston: Little, Brown, 1966.

Reuben, David. R. *Everything You Always Wanted to Know about Sex (But Were Afraid to Ask).* New York: McKay, 1969.

Smith-Lovin, Lynn, and David R. Heise. *Analyzing Social Interaction: Advances in Affect Control Theory.* New York: Gordon and Breach Science Publishers, 1988.

Stein, Martha. L. *Lovers, Friends, Slaves...The Nine Male Sexual Types.* New York: Berkley Publishing Corporation, 1974.

Stryker, Sheldon. *Symbolic Interactionism: A Social Structural Version.* Menlo Park, CA: Benjamin/Cummings, 1980.

Weiss, Michael J. *The Clustered World: How We Live, What We Buy, and What It Means about Who We Are.* Boston: Little, Brown, 2000.

Whitman, Walt. *Leaves of Grass.* Edited by David S. Reynolds. New York: Oxford University Press, 2005.

Photo Credits

Cover

Chapter 1

Exercise 1

Exercise 2

© Prodaksyn/Shutterstock.com; © Phil Date/Shutterstock.com; © Gabriela Trojanowska/Shutterstock.com; © Tarragona/Dreamstime.com; © Nick Stubbs/Dreamstime.com; © Edie Layland/ Dreamstime.com; © Tandem/Shutterstock.com; © Sophie Bengtsson/Shutterstock.com; © MichaelJung/Shutterstock.com; © Altafulla/Shutterstock.com; © Kurhan/Shutterstock.com; © Johan Geerber/Shutterstock.com

Chapter 2

Exercise 2

© Michael Hind/Shutterstock.com; © Stocksnapper/Dreamstime.com; © Sean Nel/Shutterstock.com; © Andrea Rankovic/Dreamstime.com; © Dmitriy Shironosov/Shutterstock.com; © Kirill Mikhirev/Shutterstock.com; © Lev Dolgachov/Dreamstime.com; © Yurok Aleksandrovich/Dreamstime.com; © Vgstudio/Shutterstock.com; © Aleksandr Kurganov/Dreamstime.com; © Asiana/Shutterstock.com; © Dukibu/Shutterstock.com; © George Allen Penton/Shutterstock.com

Exercise 3

© Gunnar Pippel/Shutterstock.com; © Yuri Arcurs/Dreamstime.com; © Lev Olkha/Shutterstock.com; © Ostill/Shutterstock.com; © Andrea Rankovic/Dreamstime.com; © Branislav Ostojic/Dreamstime.coml; © Oleksandr Zuyev/Dreamstime.com; © Nina Vaclavova/Dreamstime.com; © Hongqi Zhang/Dreamstime.com; © Ana Blazic/Shutterstock.com; © Sean Nel/Shutterstock.com; © Altafulla/Shutterstock.com; © Maksim Toome/Shutterstock.com; © Iurii Kryvenko/Dreamstime.com; © Sophie Phelps/Dreamstime.com

Chapter 3

Exercise 1

© Avdeev077/Dreamstime.com; © Ron Chapple Studios/Dreamstime.com; © Monkey Business Images/Dreamstime.com; © Pavel Sazonov/Shutterstock.com; © Alexey Arkhipov/Dreamstime.com; © Rmarmion/Dreamstime.com; © Yuri Arcurs/Dreamstime.com; © Lim Seng Kui/Dreamstime.com; © Rmarmion/Dreamstime.com; © Zoom Team/Shutterstock.com; © Jason Stitt/Dreamstime.com; © Ostill/Shutterstock.com; © Elena Weber/Dreamstime.com

Exercise 2

© Monkey Business Images/Dreamstime.com; © Konstantin Sutyagin/Dreamstime.com; © Katrina Brown/ Dreamstime.com; © Sean Prior/Shutterstock.com; © Pavalache Stelian/Dreamstime.com; © Markstout/Dreamstime.com; © Monika Olszewska/Shutterstock.com; © Vgstudio/Shutterstock.com; © Showface/Dreamstime.com; © Daniel76/Dreamstime.com; © Lunamarina/Dreamstime.com; © Marco Mayer/Shutterstock.com; © Miramiska/Shutterstock.com

Figures 1 and 3

© Rmarmion/Dreamstime.com; © Yuri Arcurs/Dreamstime.com; © Lim Seng Kui/Dreamstime.com; © Rmarmion/Dreamstime.com; © Zoom Team/Shutterstock.com; © Jason Stitt/Dreamstime.com; © Ostill/Shutterstock.com; © Elena Weber/Dreamstime.com

Figures 2 and 4

© Markstout/Dreamstime.com; © Monika Olszewska/Shutterstock.com; © Vgstudio/Shutterstock.com; © Showface/Dreamstime.com; © Daniel76/Dreamstime.com; © Lunamarina/Dreamstime.com; © Marco Mayer/Shutterstock.com; © Miramiska/Shutterstock.com

Chapter 6

Exercise 1

© Phil Date/Dreamstime.com; © Markusphoto/Dreamstime.com; © Ron Chapple Studios/Dreamstime.com; © Simone Van Den Berg/Dreamstime.com; © Imagez/Dreamstime.com; © Jason Stitt/Dreamstime.com; © Mtorrell/Shutterstock.com; © Coka/Shutterstock.com; © Monkey Business Images/Dreamstime.com; © Sergei Butorin/Shutterstock.com; © Lawrence Larsen/Dreamstime.com; © Kirill Mikhirev/Shutterstock.com

Exercise 2

© Iulius Costache/Dreamstime.com; © Andris Tkacenko/Dreamstime.com; © Markstout/Dreamstime.com; © Josetandem/Dreamstime.com; © Jason Stitt/Dreamstime.com; © Robert Lerich/Dreamstime.com; © Monkey Business Images/Dreamstime.com; © Francesco Cura/Dreamstime.com; © Charles Shapiro/Shutterstock.com; © Yuri Arcurs/Dreamstime.com

Chapter 7

Exercise 1

© Alexsey Fursov/Shutterstock.com; © Hunta/Shutterstock.com; © Kathy Wynn/Dreamstime.com; © Valentin Mosichev/Shutterstock.

com; © Dmitriy Melnikov/Dreamstime.com; © Viorel Sima/ Shutterstock.com; © Ostill/Shutterstock.com; © © Phartisan/ Dreamstime.com; © Bambi L. Dingman/Dreamstime.com; © Lisa F. Young/Dreamstime.com; © Jason Stitt/Shutterstock.com

Exercise 2

© Phil Date/Shutterstock.com; © Jperagine/Dreamstime.com; © Kurhan/Shutterstock.com; © Corolanty/Dreamstime.com; © Francesco Cura/Dreamstime.com; © Yuri Arcurs/Dreamstime. com; © Konstantin Sutyagin/Dreamstime.com; © ImageryMajestic/ Shutterstock.com; © Stephen Coburn/Dreamstime.com

Exercises 3 and 4

© Vgstudio/Shutterstock.com; © Petrenko Andriy/Shutterstock. com; © Vgstudio/Shutterstock.com; © Hongqi Zhang/Dreamstime. com; © MichaelJung/Shutterstock.com; © Andriy Goncharenko/ Shutterstock.com; © Yuri Arcurs/Shutterstock.com; © Lev Olkha/ Shutterstock.com; © Ivan Bliznetsov/Dreamstime.com; © Krivenko/ Shutterstock.com

Chapter 8

Exercise 1

© Sean Nel/Dreamstime.com; © Denys Dolnikov/Dreamstime. com; © Tom Nance/Shutterstock.com; © Ron Chapple Studios/ Dreamstime.com; © Yuri Arcurs/Dreamstime.com; © Sean Prior/ Shutterstock.com; © Lev Olkha/Shutterstock.com; © Diego Cervo/ Shutterstock.com; © Dmitriy Melnikov/Dreamstime.com; © Suprijono Suharjoto/Dreamstime.com

Exercise 2

© Maksim Toome/Shutterstock.com; © Diego Cervo/Shutterstock. com;©Markstout/Dreamstime.com;©AZPworldwide/Shutterstock. com; © Anatoliy Samara/Dreamstime.com; © Tarragona/ Dreamstime.com; © Monika Olszewska/Shutterstock.com; © Maksim Toome/Shutterstock.com; © Lev Olkha/Shutterstock.com; © Sean Nel/Shutterstock.com; © Stephanie Swartz/Dreamstime. com; © Andresr/Shutterstock.com

Exercise 3

© Soundsnaps/Shutterstock.com; © Sam Robles/Shutterstock. com; © Jeff Walthall/Dreamstime.com; © Anthony Aneese Totah Jr/Dreamstime.com; © Gino Santa Maria/Dreamstime.com; © Lee Prince/Shutterstock.com; © Photosani/Shutterstock.com; © MichaelJung/Shutterstock.com; © Modi1980/Dreamstime.com; © Vitalii Nesterchuk/Shutterstock.com; © Andrey Burmakin/ Shutterstock.com; © Pichugin Dmitry/Shutterstock.com; © Biancoloto/Shutterstock.com; © Tandem/Shutterstock.com; © SipaPhoto/Shutterstock.com; © Kendy/Shutterstock.com

Chapter 9

Exercise 1

© Warren Goldswain/Shutterstock.com; © Jason Stitt/Dreamstime. com; © Mark Stout Photography/Shutterstock.com; © Christopher Howey/Dreamstime.com; © Wallenrock/Shutterstock.com; © Boumen&Japet/Shutterstock.com; © Margarita Borodina/ Shutterstock.com; © RJ Lerich/Shutterstock.com; © Avava/ Shutterstock.com; © Zuijeta/Shutterstock.com; © Sophie Louise Phelps/Shutterstock.com; © Istvan Csak/Shutterstock.com; © Jurate Lasiene/Shutterstock.com; © Maga/Shutterstock.com

Exercise 2

© Netbritish/Shutterstock.com; © Stryjek/Shutterstock.com; © Termit/Shutterstock.com; © Aaleksander/Dreamstime.com; © Bliznetsov/Shutterstock.com; © Deklofenak/Shutterstock.com; © Stephen Orsillo/Shutterstock.com; © Lana K/Shutterstock.com; © AZPworldwide/Shutterstock.com; © Jason Stitt/Shutterstock.com; © Zdenka Darula/Dreamstime.com; © Newphotoservice/Shutterstock.com; © Elena Elfimova/Shutterstock.com; © Sergei Butorin/Shutterstock.com; © Magicnfoto/Shutterstock.com; © Gansovsky Vladislav/Dreamstime.com

Exercise 3

© Tyler Olson/Shutterstock.com; © Vgstudio/Shutterstock.com; © Karin Hildebrand Lau/Shutterstock.com; © Kurhan/Shutterstock.com; © Jacqueline Abromeit/Shutterstock.com; © Tomasz Trojanowski/Shutterstock.com; © Warren Goldswain/Shutterstock.com; © PDImages/Shutterstock.com; © Dmitriy Shironosov/Shutterstock.com; © Eastwest Imaging/Dreamstime.com; © Navita/Shutterstock.com; © Polushkina Svetlana/Shutterstock.com; © Altafulla/Shutterstock.com; © Kiselev Andrey Valerevich/Shutterstock.com; © Prodaksyn/Shutterstock.com; © Iofoto/Shutterstock.com

Chapter 10

Exercise 1

© Simone Van Den Berg/Dreamstime.com; © Jason Stitt/Shutterstock.com; © Theodor38/Dreamstime.com; © Paulbuceta/Dreamstime.com; © Ron Chapple Studios/Dreamstime.com; © AXL/Shutterstock.com; © Simone Van Den Berg/Dreamstime.com; © Jason Stitt/Dreamstime.com; © Duard Van Der Westhuizen/

Dreamstime.com; © Laurent Hamels/Dreamstime.com; © Yuri Acrurs/Shutterstock.com; © Ipatov/Shutterstock.com; © Paul Moore/Dreamstime.com; © Carlo Dapino/Dreamstime.com

Exercise 2

© Shawn Werner/Dreamstime.com; © Zdenka Darula/Dreamstime.com; © Timur Grigoryev/Dreamstime.com; © Robert Lerich/Dreamstime.com; © Jason Stitt/Dreamstime.com; © Miroslav Georgijevic/Dreamstime.com; © Andres Rodriguez/Dreamstime.com; © Markstout/Dreamstime.com; © Steven Pepple/Dreamstime.com; © Showface/Dreamstime.com; © Christopher Howey/Dreamstime.com; © David Davis/Dreamstime.com; © Tissiana/Dreamstime.com; © Gabriela Trojanowska/Shutterstock.com

Exercises 3 and 4

© David Davis/Dreamstime.com; © Ipatov/Shutterstock.com; © Christopher Howey/Dreamstime.com; © Yuri Acrurs/Shutterstock.com; © Markstout/Dreamstime.com; © Jason Stitt/Dreamstime.com; © Andres Rodriguez/Dreamstime.com; © Simone Van Den Berg/Dreamstime.com; © Gabriela Trojanowska/Shutterstock.com; © Carlo Dapino/Dreamstime.com; © Paul Moore/Dreamstime.com; © Showface/Dreamstime.com; © Duard Van Der Westhuizen/Dreamstime.com; © Steven Pepple/Dreamstime.com; © Laurent Hamels/Dreamstime.com; © Rmarmion/Dreamstime.com; © Lim Seng Kui/Dreamstime.com; © Rmarmion/Dreamstime.com; © Zoom Team/Shutterstock.com; © Ostill/Shutterstock.com; © Elena Weber/Dreamstime.com; © Monika Olszewska/Shutterstock.com; © Vgstudio/Shutterstock.com; © Daniel76/Dreamstime.com; © Lunamarina/Dreamstime.com; © Marco Mayer/Shutterstock.com; © Miramiska/Shutterstock.com

Figures 1 and 3

© Simone Van Den Berg/Dreamstime.com; © Jason Stitt/ Dreamstime.com; © Duard Van Der Westhuizen/Dreamstime.com; © Laurent Hamels/Dreamstime.com; © Yuri Acrurs/Shutterstock. com; © Ipatov/Shutterstock.com; © Paul Moore/Dreamstime.com; © Carlo Dapino/Dreamstime.com

Figures 2 and 4

© Andres Rodriguez/Dreamstime.com; © Markstout/Dreamstime. com; © Steven Pepple/Dreamstime.com; © Showface/Dreamstime. com; © Christopher Howey/Dreamstime.com; © David Davis/ Dreamstime.com; © Tissiana/Dreamstime.com; © Gabriela Trojanowska/Shutterstock.com

Chapter 11

Exercise 3

© Simone Van Den Berg/Dreamstime.com; © Jason Stitt/Dreamstime. com; © Duard Van Der Westhuizen/Dreamstime.com; © Laurent Hamels/Dreamstime.com; © Yuri Acrurs/Shutterstock.com; © Ipatov/Shutterstock.com; © Paul Moore/Dreamstime.com; © Carlo Dapino/Dreamstime.com; © Andres Rodriguez/Dreamstime.com; © Markstout/Dreamstime.com; © Steven Pepple/Dreamstime.com; © Showface/Dreamstime.com; © Christopher Howey/Dreamstime. com; © David Davis/Dreamstime.com; © Tissiana/Dreamstime. com; © Gabriela Trojanowska/Shutterstock.com

Exercise 4

© Yuri Acurs/Shutterstock.com; © Jason Stitt/Shutterstock.com; © Sean Nel/Shutterstock.com

Exercise 5

© Diana Lundin/Dreamstime.com; © Francesco Cura/Dreamstime. com; © Sakir N/Shutterstock.com

Figures 1 and 2

© Simone Van Den Berg/Dreamstime.com; © Jason Stitt/ Dreamstime.com; © Duard Van Der Westhuizen/Dreamstime.com; © Laurent Hamels/Dreamstime.com; © Yuri Acrurs/Shutterstock. com; © Ipatov/Shutterstock.com; © Paul Moore/Dreamstime.com; © Carlo Dapino/Dreamstime.com

About the Author

Mark Thompson, PhD, is a clinical psychologist, researcher, and Internet pioneer. He helped design matchmaking systems for the two largest online dating websites, Yahoo! and Match.com. His interactive tests on physical attraction, personality types, sexual adventurousness, and love styles have been taken by over thirty million people worldwide. Dr. Thompson has published articles on social psychology, interpersonal relationships, public health, and healthcare reform. This is his first book. He invites you to join the conversation about the book and take a free interactive test at www.whoshouldyouhavesexwith.com.